From Bombs to Babies

A Memoir

ISBN: 1453741720
EAN-13: 9781453741726
LCCN: 2010911735

From Bombs to Babies

A Memoir

R.L.Rackliffe

TABLE OF CONTENTS

*Dedicated to: **Dr. George D. Radford***

*To tell how I fulfilled a promise we made to each other
on a jungle road on Saipan in the spring of 1945
during the war against Japan.*

PREFACE

"What a coincidence" is an expression used by all of us whenever we learn of something—a person, a situation, an event—that we have experienced ourselves or shared with others. But what of the coincidences that make you sit up and ask yourself, *how did that happen?* One or two in a lifetime we can understand, but many, very many, over a lifetime that always place you in a position you could only dream of seems strange.

In looking back over my not inconsiderable time on this earth and chronicling events from my teens right up to present day, I began to realize what power had influenced my decisions, the people I met, the places I visited, enabling me to be in the right place at the right time and helping others get through seemingly impossible situations.

Starting out in New England, with all the twists and turns of family life, the strict upbringing brought deep frustrations, the inexplicable actions of a father, and the friendships that led to eventually gaining my independence as a physician.

This is the true story of an ordinary man finding himself in extra ordinary situations: discovering an ability to cure coupled with an intense, and very real, sense of direction coming from you will have to read this story to find out what.

From being stationed on Saipan during WWII with the first B-29 outfit based in the Marianas, dropping bombs on Japan, to working in Haiti with the nuns in one of Mother Theresa's homes—this is my story, full of love, life, danger, and excitement. It's an unbelievable journey, not without laughter and tears, joy and sadness. Prepare yourself for a rollercoaster ride and find out what really happened. Ask yourself if you can explain -why- there is really only one viable answer.

All the events described are true, but the names of some have been changed to protect their privacy.

PART 1:

EARLY YEARS TO WWII

M y first recollection in my life is one of loss. My mother said, "Sarah isn't going to be with us anymore."

We three children (my sister Janet, my brother Foster, and I) had lived with Sarah; we had eaten all our meals with her. She was my mother to me; she had changed my diapers, dressed me in the mornings, and undressed me and tucked me in at night.. She had wiped away my tears and loved me. And she had cried the last night she was with us, so I got up in her lap and helped her cry. She was my mother, until that day when I was three or four and she walked away.

The day she left, Mother didn't go out; she stayed home all day. She had never done this before. Usually she disappeared for the day, and Sarah took care of us. Mother called her our nursemaid, but to me, Sarah was my mother. Dad said that we couldn't afford her anymore. The year was 1927. My father, who had dazzled the city with his quick rise to wealth, had built two large apartment complexes on Glen Street in New Britain. He had also worked in the family business, Rackliffe Bros. Co., Incorporated, a sprawling enterprise that claimed an entire city block. There was an enormous hardware store, mill supply, sash and door division, and an agricultural division that handled all International Harvester machinery and parts for the entire Hartford County. There was a fleet of six trucks delivering sash and door, farm machinery, mill supplies, and hardware all over the state.

In addition, my father Fredric O. Rackliffe served two terms in the state legislature before 1927, the year he was thirty-one.

By that year the economy was in a downslide, heading towards the stock market crash of 1929, and people who had rented my father's apartments could no longer afford them.

Ultimately, he lost everything he had except for the family business that his father and his father's brothers had started. Rackliffe Bros. had a sound financial position in contrast to his own apartments, which had been much more speculative, and therefore, shaky—a much more risky financial undertaking.

In 1924, while in the legislature, he was asked by Senator Fred Walcott who was going to run for governor of the state to join him and run for lieutenant governor.

While considering this, he received a letter warning him that if he ran for lieutenant governor, I would be exposed as the bastard son of our family doctor. I learned when I was in my early teens that this became a standing joke between the two families, and I was often called "Dr. Mike" when the adults were together.

All four of us children were born at home, with my father assisting Dr. Mike at the deliveries. When the delivery was due, Dr. Mike would sleep at the house.

At any rate, Dad did not run for lieutenant governor. I think he was just too busy.

He built a grandiose home next to my grandfather's 1800s house, on land that was originally part of my grandfather's farm.

With Sarah gone, Mother showed us love and dropped out of her former social life completely to take care of us. My father assumed more and more control of the business as my grandfather aged.

In 1928, my brother Don was born, and when he was five, he joined us at the dining room table for dinner every night. He sat next to Mom on my right. Probably because Mom came from wealth, dinner was always formal; linen table cloth and napkins, polished silver napkin rings, and always four candles in silver candlesticks. As we sat at the table, I was at my father's right, with him at one end of the table and Mom at the other. Foster and Janet sat opposite Donald and me.

At about that time I was seven years old; my father really began to make me his whipping boy. I never found out why, but it was terrible to bear, because I loved him, and it hurt like hell to have him mad at me.

At dinner time, the family would no sooner be seated than he would start nagging me relentlessly, calling me names. "Flannel mouth" was his favorite, and he would just keep correcting me; ridiculing me incessantly until I was in tears. If I asked to be excused, he would deny the request. Often I would look down at Mother (for help I guess), and she would be sitting there silently with tears running down her face.

There were times too when he really knocked me around. Once, he knocked me right over a chair in the air because I didn't want to wear some knickers my mother had set out for me.

After he had finished with me, we were ordered into the family car, which was a coupe with a rumble seat. We three sat in the rumble seat, and Donald rode on Mom's lap inside. We were heading for the shore, so that Mom could visit with friends while Dad played golf.

Following that beating I was mad as hell, so I refused to talk at all on the way down and until Dad had left for his golf game. As we were getting in the car for the homeward trip, Dad took me by the shoulder and said: "I played awful today, and it was because of you."

That pleased me, so as I climbed into the rumble seat in between Foster and Jan, I smiled. I was happy I had ruined his day. He sure had done a number on mine.

My best friend in my whole life was my brother Foster. He and Janet would sit at the table while Dad was working me over and say nothing, but look down at their plates.

Fos and I never had a fight, even though we were always together. We played tennis in a court in our back yard constantly (Foster had a wicked cut shot that used to infuriate me while he stood at the net and laughed).

He was indisputably my dad's favorite and was expected to succeed him in the business. It was a given. I was happy with that because from the time I was seven or eight, I wanted to be a doctor.

Every Christmas there was always a really nice bunch of toys for Foster, while my gifts were never much except for clothing. But Foster always shared his toys with me so it didn't matter. At age fourteen, I got a bicycle because he had suggested it to my dad. The bicycle had been in the store for over a year or so, and it didn't look as though it was going to sell anyway.

The bastard story was told laughingly to me in my teens by my father. I said nothing, but it explained his attitude and behavior toward me, why he didn't run for lieutenant governor, and my mother's tears.

When he was wealthy, Dad had set up funds for education for three of us, and I will never forget signing my stock certificates so that Foster could go to a military school (like my dad had done), and Janet could go to the University of New Hampshire.

We didn't go on any vacations because we couldn't afford them, but the grove behind my grandfather's house was really a vacation for all during the Depression.

At the age of fourteen, I applied for a job as kitchen helper at a camp in Maine. I got the job on my own, and then told my parents what I was going to be doing that summer. They did not object, so from then on I arranged my own summers.

The next year I was a counselor in the cadet (youngest kids) division of Camp Woodstock. I helped six boys that summer, and it made me feel great. Nearly all the boys came to this camp for a two-week period, so every two weeks there would be lots of good byes in the morning, and greeting of newcomers in the afternoon.

As they unloaded, every now and then a new camper would have four to six blankets with him, and the parent would say, "Jimmy wets the bed, so he'll need a blanket change. He is going to stay for one month unless he doesn't like it."

Well, I figured they wouldn't last a week once the kids in the cabin knew. It brought back some rough experiences to me. Both my sister and I were bed wetters, and I remember one summer when I was ten, I sat on my chair as punishment every morning all summer at the shore, while the kids would call me "Stinky," and taunt me from the lawn outside the window.

I made up my mind that no kid in my cabin was going to go through that embarrassment and feeling of shame. I got them up twice a night to void.

Nobody went home early.

The next year I had the whole junior division; six cabins with six counselors under me, and while we had boys come in with the large piles of blankets, we scored a perfect one hundred keeping the kids dry.

How their personalities changed as the stigma was erased! They were like flower buds that came into bloom. Their joy and happiness made the whole camp a happier place.

I was so happy for them! I loved them, and they loved me back.

My last year at camp was 1941. I had the junior division again. In the second two-week period, a ten-year-old boy named Alan was one of the campers. His mother pulled me aside and told me, "Alan's dad died suddenly six months ago, so I don't know how this is going to be for him. Please give him special attention, and if you think he isn't happy, please call me."

"Don't worry about a thing. Count on me. I'll call if I need to." I looked at him standing there by his bunk, a beautiful, perfectly formed ten-year-old boy, standing erect and composed. He had blonde hair and beautiful big blue eyes, with a smile that tore my heart out. I felt so bad for him! I loved him from the start, and for the time that he was there, I tried to be a father to him. His time at camp was wonderful for him. The day he was leaving, I promised to write to him every week, and before he got into the car, he turned with tears in his eyes and hugged me tightly.

"I love you, Alan, and I'll be in touch. You can count on it."

As they drove away, I got a little teary myself.

I stuck to my word and wrote him every week. During the fall, I visited with him on weekends.

One weekend I took Alan to New York City, where we stayed at the Sloan House (YMCA).

We did the automat and the Statue of Liberty, and just had a great weekend together. We also went to the top of the Empire State Building.

Alan's mom invited me up for the first weekend in December. That Sunday was December 7, 1941, and we listened in disbelief as the Japanese attacked Pearl Harbor. As I said goodbye that evening, I wondered if I would ever see Alan again.

Looking back, I realize I was trying to act like I thought a father should act for Alan.

It was during this period that my dad and I began to enjoy each other's company. It all started when I was about fourteen. My father was invited by one of his business acquaintances to go down to Yale's Woolsey Hall to hear the evangelist E. Stanley Jones. Dad took me along. Now my father never went to church and had very little interest in religion until that night. At the end of his inspirational sermon, Mr. Jones invited all the men in that great hall to come forward, be baptized again, and commit their lives to Christ. To my surprise, my father got up and joined the crowd going up to the front of the hall. The music from the massive organ made the rededication all the more impressive. Dad was quiet all the way home, and I learned later that at two in the morning he woke up our pastor by throwing pebbles against his bedroom window. When the pastor stuck out his head, he asked,: "Who is it? And what do you want?"

"It's Fred Rackliffe, and I've come to serve Jesus."

"Well, go home and call me at ten in the morning." The window shut.

At ten the next morning my father called the pastor, they met at the church, and Reverend Bovee smiled at my father and said: "God has been listening to me and you are the answer he has sent me to take over the high school class. We have over fifty of them in the church and yet only have about six to ten in Sunday school." My father accepted the challenge and in one year he had the attendance up in the high forties. If someone didn't show up for class, he got a phone call enquiring as to why he wasn't there. He ran that class for twenty years. I still meet people who were in it who comment on what a great influence it was for them—and that was fifty years ago!

From that day on, he became an acting Christian, and along with that, our relationship improved by leaps and bounds.

He was just a great guy, and I enjoyed and admired him. He had a personality that took the air out of a room when he entered, with a firm full voice and a hearty laugh and handshake that won people over to him with ease.

And he was a talented pianist. One summer on a beautiful Sunday, Mr. and Mrs. Hardy Payor came to visit. They were great friends of my folks, and Hardy and my father were perfect for each other; dynamic and talented, pretty much equals at the piano.

When Hardy saw the grand piano and the upright piano in the living room, he hooted: "Come on, Fred, get out some music, and let's play!' He seated himself at the upright, and while waiting for my father to produce the sheet music, bedazzled everyone with beautiful runs of music and grand chords. Dad handed out several sheets of music of which he had duplicates and they agreed on a piece by Rachmaninoff, "Vocalise." After a few bad starts, they got in synch and the music was beautiful. It filled the room and flowed out the open windows to the front yard and the street.

They were both superb pianists, and they enjoyed the accompanying piano and the interplay between them became more polished and natural as they continued to play. After an hour or so, there were about five to ten people listening in the front yard. when they finished with the "War of 1812" by Tchaikovsky, applause erupted from the listening neighbors. It was an event to cherish.

While I was in high school, my folks lost their house. They simply could not make the mortgage payments during the Depression, so they arranged to move back with my grandparents, whose house was next door.

Foster and I each got our friends together and six to eight of us moved every single piece of furniture from a ten-room-house over to my grandparents' home. We walked the stuff over, everything from cellar to attic except the refrigerator and stove.

My father went off on a business trip when we started the move and did not come home until the job was done. That had to be hard on him.

In September 1941, dad told me that the "driver of the 'city truck'" was leaving and said, "You can have the job."

"Okay, Dad. Thanks."

Henry Fairwood was the man who was leaving for a job with a more promising future. He was a nice guy, and he stayed on and rode with me for the first week to show me the routes and tricks at the different factories that we serviced. He also gave me tips on who to avoid, when to make certain calls, and to count on everything being correct when Jack Arrowsmith, the shipping clerk, said it was.

Finally, Henry was gone, and I became the city truck driver for Rackliffe Bros. on my own.

With the war going very badly in early 1942, it was a very sad day when my brother Foster left to join the USAAF. The morning after he left, Bob Steele's radio program was on as I got ready to go to work. They played "My Buddy," which hit me right between the eyes, as I looked at Foster's unused bed. I cried all the way through that song, standing there looking at the unused bed as I thought of him.

The thought of the new job got me out of the teary mood and headed me down to breakfast with Mom.

Mom had made me a "sandwich spread" sandwich in a brown bag along with a couple of cookies for my lunch. I slugged down my coffee, gave her a peck on the cheek, and flew down the back stairs, two at a time to my truck, which was parked under the sickle pear tree in the back yard.

It was a neat green '41 Ford half ton pick up and with an eight cylinder engine, it could really haul ass!

I was at the store in about ten minutes. After parking outside of shipping and receiving, I went in to greet my boss, Jack Arrowsmith.

Jack had been employed by Rackliffe Bros. since his arrival in the 1920s from England, and a more proper Englishman has never existed. He had served twenty years in the British Army before being mustered out and was alleged to have told the Prince of Wales to put his cigar out because he was in a no smoking area. The law was the law to Jack, and he didn't back down.

After his discharge, he and his wife Lucy emigrated to the states and to New Britain, where my grandfather hired him as shipping and receiving clerk.

He was a fastidious person. His face glowed from scrubbing; his hair had a little curl in the front that was never out of place.

He wore a clean shirt every day and had garters around his arms to keep the cuffs at the proper level. He was married to his pipe, which rarely left his mouth all day. The pipe made him look like his chin stuck out, which gave him a look of determination. He was the personification of the British bulldog. His favorite saying, which I shall never forget, was, "Always leave a clean edge."

I loved working for him. We started working together in September of 1941 and by 1942, I was an old hand. He was such a straight shooter and everything had to be done just right. The longer we worked together, the less he supervised me. One day in April when I got there for the morning, he greeted me and gestured toward a pile of packages, already wrapped and ready to go. The pipe came out of the mouth. "Morning, Bob." He pointed his pipe to the corner where there were several items stacked. "That pile over there is your first load. You'd better start at Skinner Precision industries; there are some mill supply items in their order that they are waiting for."

"Okay, Jack." I started out, figuring the most efficient route starting at Skinner's, and loaded my truck.

I gave Jack my itinerary in case he had to call me, and headed out the door.

"See you about noon, Jack."

By 11:35, I was heading back from Southington to New Britain for a break and lunch. I parked outside

Shipping and Receiving, and brought in the receipts to Jack.

"Hello, Bob," he said as I entered and gave him the receipts. "There was a phone call for you from a Mr. Barnes at the 'Y.' He wants you to call him at your convenience."

"Thanks, Jack. I'll call him right away."

Mr. Barnes was the general secretary of the New Britain YMCA. I got to know him in 1940—1941 when the "Y" formed neighborhood boys' clubs. These developed during the Depression as part of a city-wide project. Each club received a pass to swim and use the gym free, one day a week. There were more than ten clubs set up in the city, covering the residential areas completely. My club was in the southern part of the city and was composed of twenty youngsters, age eight to eleven, whose enthusiasm for any kind of adventure was unbounded. They named the club the "Rinkydinks."

I spent a lot of my weekends with the Rinkydinks. We would go on hikes every weekend, and each week they got to use the "Y" facilities free. Almost every weekend, we were off hiking the nearby open spaces.

On many occasions, we camped for the weekend in the grove behind our house, setting up tents in a circle, and cooking on the fireplace that was located there.

I assumed that Mr. Barnes wanted to talk to me about my Rinkydinks, so I called his office and made an appointment for 5:00 p.m. the next day.

The YMCA building had been built in the late 1800s and faced out on the southwest corner of Central Park in downtown New Britain. The building was made of huge brownstone blocks. The ground floor was occupied by two clothing stores—one for men, and one for ladies. It was on the corner of Court and Main streets.

To its left was a grand Civil War Memorial that stood thirty feet high, with a huge eagle, in flight, on the peak in Central Park. At the south end of the park, there were subterranean restrooms for both ladies and gentlemen. At the south end of Central Park, with its spire reaching toward God, was the South Congregational Church (also made of Brownstone blocks). Its carillon playing at weekday noon times and on Sundays was enjoyed by all those who happened to be downtown. The music conveyed an air of permanence and peace. As I hurried toward the "Y" for my meeting with Mr. Barnes, I passed this entire beautiful and familiar scene. I had a feeling of belonging.

The entrance to the "Y" was on Court Street and had an open brownstone stairway going up one flight to the men's section. Inside the men's floor, there was another set of stairs up to the boys' section.

The men's floor had a gym and some handball courts, while the boys' floor had a gym and a marble pool, which was about forty feet long, thirty feet wide, and six feet deep at one end. Both the men and the boys used it. Bathing was nude, which was a problem for some of the boys, but being in a group helped them to overcome any self-consciousness. It puzzled me as to why they ever decided to put the pool on the third floor.

As I doubled up the stairs to the men's section, heading towards Mr. Barnes's office, I wondered what was up. I knocked on his door, and was told to come in by the voice of Mr. Barnes. I pushed open the door and entered. He was sitting at his desk, looking at me as I came in.

"Hi, Mr. Barnes, did you want to see me?"

"Yes, I did, Bob. Have a seat." As he gestured towards a chair.

I sat down facing him across his desk. He looked straight at my eyes through his rimless glasses, his hands folded on the desk in front of him wearing a slight smile on his face. He said, "Bob, how'd you like to go to college?"

"I can't afford it, sir—"

He held up his hand to stop me from talking, and when I stopped and looked at him, he said in a very emphatic tone, "Bob, you are bright. You have more to offer.

You need to consider this offer. College will make a big difference in your life. You've been working for your father for over a year now. You should go to college. A local businessman has offered to pay your tuition. The only provision is that you have to repay it, without interest, as soon as you can, so another deserving person can have the same opportunity. What do you think?"

"Who is the businessman, Mr. Barnes?"

"He prefers to be anonymous, because he already has six young men in college on loans such as yours."

I was dumbfounded. I had given up any idea of doing anything except working in the family business along with my older brother Foster. Now there was a door in front of me with "Doctor" on it. This seemed so impossible, but there it was: an opportunity in the road that said: "Turn here."

I thanked Mr. Barnes and the unnamed donor and accepted the offer. I never thought it would happen after Dad's apartment buildings were lost. With the further loss of the money put way for education, the idea of going to college seemed far out of reach. Now out of the blue, there was a way I could start on the road I had always dreamed of. I was ecstatic! I decided to make my announcement at dinner that night.

As the four of us sat down to dinner (Janet had married and was living in Ohio, and Foster was in Miami Beach in the Air Force Officers Candidate School), I made the announcement proudly.

"Mom and Dad, Mr. Barnes called me in today and has offered me a full tuition scholarship at Springfield College. Isn't that neat? I'll be starting in the fall!"

Mom looked at me in amazement. Her face broke into a huge smile. "That's wonderful, Bobbie! I am so happy for you."

"It's an interest free scholarship for the full tuition. The man who is giving them has six going at one time. All I have to do is pay it back as soon as possible, so that someone else can have a chance. "

Dad asked, "Who is this man?"

"Mr. Barnes said he does not want to have his identity known, so I don't know who he is."

Mom said, turning to my dad, "What a wonderful thing to do, isn't it, dear?"

His answer was like a glass of cold water being thrown in my face. "Well that's just great! Fred Rackliffe's boy is being given a charity donation to go to college because his father can't afford it!" He stared at me angrily like I was his bastard son, then he got up and left the dining room. I felt bad watching him go but, in retrospect, I could understand how that must have made him feel.

Watching him go, Mother took my hand in hers and said, "I think it's wonderful, Bobby, and I'm proud of you. Never mind your father, honey; he's had a bad week."

When September came around, Mom helped me get some clothes dry-cleaned, and helped me pack the laundry box she had bought for me. The last thing she put in was a package of her famous cookies.

"I'm going to miss you, Bobbie; you were always the only one to help me with the dishes at night. I'm glad you are going though—it's the right thing for you."

Dad's response was to take no interest in my going and not to help at all. On the day I was leaving for college, by bus, he came up to me as I was packing to leave and said, "Good luck, son." Then he smiled and added, "Keep your mouth shut and study hard." He then shook my hand and left for work.

That felt better.

I took the bus to Springfield (Massachusetts) College from New Britain, Connecticut and carried my belongings in the laundry box my mom had provided, along with stamps to ship my dirty clothes home for her to clean and send back (always with a surprise in the box.

At age nineteen, I registered at the college on the 15th of September in the administrative office, which was in the Old Dorm. During the sign-in I saw all the papers the college had on file for me, including a check for the tuition made out to Springfield College, signed by Sam Davidson, a very successful merchant with two stores in New Britain.

So Mr. Davidson was my benefactor!

To aid me in paying for my room and board, the college had arranged a job for me at the Brooks Bank Note Company from 6:00 to 11:00 p.m. Monday through Friday. The job was operating a big machine that cut out beer labels. I was required to place the cutting tool precisely over the stack of labels before the machine pulled the stack in and pressed the cutting tool through the two-inch stack of labels.

The Old Dorm was really old. It had ivy-covered brick walls, which were very dark, and the old wooden floors squeaked when you walked on them. The gymnasium and its aquarium, and the library were similar in age and appearance, all three having been built circa 1900.

There was a large tree-covered lawn, surrounded on three sides by these buildings. A lake glistened behind the old dorm, while at its left the New Dorm stood out in proud contrast.

It was a building of the modern era, and contained all the classrooms in the basement and on the first floor, with beautiful dorm rooms on the top two floors.

My roommate was a sullen person from Cape Cod, whose name I can't remember. He sat at his desk in the room smoking cigarettes, bitching about the food and ridiculing the school, his classes, and anything else that happened to come up. He took great pride in his ability to fart loudly and belch almost at will. To him, the louder the fart and the longer the belch, the more it pleased him. They were little sonic victories in his day.

Soon I had made friends with Charlie Stone and Hank Leete. Charlie was the son of a black minister from Philadelphia, and Hank's father was a professor at Amherst. We became inseparable.

Because we all were draft eligible, the college recommended that we join either the Naval or Army reserve, as both of these services were allowing their college reservists to stay in college in 1942, rather than call them up to active duty. Many of us joined the Army reserve.

Launching myself on a pre-med program, I struggled for four to six weeks. The chemistry and biology were like a foreign language to me. I finally admitted to myself that these subjects were way beyond me! I quickly switched majors to a Bachelor of Arts in social studies, which would qualify me to become a Boys' Work Secretary for the YMCA. Sloughing off in high school had left me totally unprepared and ignorant of how to study.

In the spring of 1943, the services established college programs and called up the reserves (us). Effectively, this closed certain colleges to civilians. The intent of the service programs was to ensure the continued education of the future generation. The Navy program was called V-1, while the Army program was labeled ASTP, which stood for Army Specialized Training Program. Both took over colleges completely, excluding all other students.

PART 2:

WAR IN THE PACIFIC

S pringfield College became a V-1 training center for the Navy. This prompted the call up of
all the Army reservists, thus clearing the campus and the facilities for the Navy. Accordingly, all
the Army reservists marched off to Camp Devens to
begin active duty and probable assignment to continue in the ASTP program at one of the colleges
taken over by the Army.

All the way to Devens, Charlie and I sat together on
the train and had a great old time kidding with the
guys around us. The war was going so badly that there
was no anger on anyone's part at having been called
up. In fact, everyone expected it and was ready to do
his part.

"I wonder if we'll end up together," Charlie said. "I'd
sure like to get in the Aviation Cadets."

"Yeah, that would be great," I answered, "but I'm color-blind, so that does it for me." We continued the small
talk and laughter all the way to the camp

When we disembarked and marched into the camp, Charlie, my dear black friend, my best friend at college, was singled out and sent to another part of the camp. This was my first experience with racial segregation, and it infuriated me, but there was nothing I could do.

That day all of us from Springfield College and reservists from other colleges entered a large building and were subjected to the most dehumanizing, loud, organized, robotic, demeaning treatment, from which we emerged with a headful of orders, advice, humiliation, and a bagful of army clothes.

We wound our way through a huge room. A soldier ordered us to get into single file and, "Take off all your clothes except your skivvies. Keep moving behind the guy in front of you."

We were standing in our jockey shorts in a line alongside a table that went the length of the room. On the other side of that table were soldiers in fatigues, and behind them were all the supplies, so as we went down that line, clothing and equipment was coming at us non stop.

First, we were given cards on which to print the address of the place we wanted our clothes to go. Then all our civilian clothes were taken from us as the line kept moving. Having lost my clothes, I was ordered to step onto a device to measure foot size. As I stood on the sizing machine, a soldier handed me two pails of sand, which broadened my feet from the extra weight. He then looked at the size on the machine and shouted, "Nine and a half double eddies!" Two pairs of army boots were plunked in my arms. Nine and a half double eddies.

With shoes in hand, I moved down the line as item after item was hurled at me in quick succession.

Underwear (olive drab boxers), then fatigues (two pair), winter uniform and summer uniforms, mess kit, canteen, and lastly a duffel bag in which to put it all.

Clutching my bag of clothes and shoes and wearing fatigues for the first time, I followed the guy in front of me into a small auditorium. There we were subjected to "training films," each about twenty minutes long, covering such subjects as military rules and regulations, how to salute, how to stand at attention, how to put on a gas mask, and lastly, women and the venereal diseases they carried, even though they "looked clean."

At the end of this movie, the lights came on, and the guy in charge asked, "Does anyone have a driver's license?" Instantly, a host of arms went up, and one guy in the front was picked out.

"All right, soldier, hop up here on the stage and stand on that table so the men in the back can see." The man did as he was told.

"Now men, our volunteer here is going to demonstrate a Short Arm inspection. Pay attention. Every month you will be doing this while you are in the army, so, get it right."

Turning to the soldier on the table, he ordered him to lower his pants and underwear. After this was done he ordered the man to pull back the foreskin of his penis and then to strip it down to the glans.

When the poor bastard had complied, one of the guys from Springfield shouted out: "Let's give him three cheers!"

The embarrassed man got down off the table with a rueful smile, while the cheers rang out in the hall.

Rule #1: Never volunteer for anything—ever, ever!

Next, I entered a room crowded with desks, each with a chair by the side, facing the person at the desk.

At this station, I was given the financial side of things. Who did I want to name as beneficiary on my life insurance? What did I want to do with my monthly pay?

I sent a large portion of my pay to my father, asking him to pay off the loan for college, first by giving the money to Mr. Barnes, and then open a bank account for me. I wanted to build a nest egg for my education when I returned.

One day while at Devens, I was pulled for KP duty. Arriving at the mess hall at 5:00 a.m., my first job was to peel potatoes and cut them up for the supper meal. They plopped a bushel bag full of potatoes in front of me, along with four five-gallon pots. It took me and two others until noon or thereabouts to fill those four pots.

At 2:00 p.m., I was assigned a new job: to place all the salt and pepper shakers on each table, in line with those on all other tables. They had to be in line at zero degrees and ninety degrees no exceptions. This idiocy took the remainder of the afternoon.

The next day a group of us was shipped to the Air Force in Miami Beach. When we disembarked from the train, we were divided into squadrons and taken by truck to the hotels on Collins Avenue. All the hotels had been taken over by the U.S. Army Air Force, and were used as the basic training center for the USAAF.

It was here that we first met our drill instructor, a cocky son of a bitch named Sergeant D'Amico, who for the next six weeks would torment us, ridicule us, punish us, and literally run our lives.

He showed us how he wanted the beds made so tight that a quarter would bounce when dropped on the blanket. shoes were to be shined and lined up under the bed—toes out at exactly the edge of the frame of the bed. The lobby floor was to be scrubbed every day as punishment for whatever he chose to object to, and, "If it isn't clean, you'll be down here on your hands and knees scrubbing it with your tooth brush!"

He was one tough, nasty son of a bitch.

Every day for six weeks, we were out on Collins Avenue, along with thousands of other recruits, marching up and down that hotel-lined street. It was like singing in a canyon, as the singing reverberated off the concrete walls formed by the hotels along the entire length of Collins Avenue.

It was a dramatic scene, with hundreds of squadrons all marching on the same street, singing different tunes loudly, in perfect step. The sound of thousands of men singing and marching was an awesome spectacle. Standing in one place and hearing and seeing the troops march by made the songs blend into one another as they came down the street, and then faded away as they went by. It was truly inspiring.

Every squadron marching along was singing a different song, so that if a person stood still and listened as the squadrons marched by the effect was like this: "Wait 'til the SUN SHINES NELLIE AND THE clouds go drifting by—around her neck she wore a yellow RIBBON AND IF YOU ASKED HER why the hell she wore it—off we go into the wild blue yonder AT 'EM BOYS GIVE HER THE GUN here they come zooming to—roll out the barrel WE'LL HAVE A BARREL OF FUN sing boom ta rara—John Brown's body lies a MOLDING IN HIS GRAVE John brown's body lies a molding in his grave—underneath the lamppost by the village gate, fare thee well LILLY MARLENE, FARE THEE WELL LILLY Marlene—"

The effect was spine chilling: each song getting to a crescendo as they went by, then fading into the distance as the next song demanded increasing attention, while marching stridently towards the stationary listener.

While doing all this singing, we learned to march with precision: to about face, march on an oblique, to the right flank, to the left flank, and to the rear march, all in step and while singing.

From sunup to taps our DI (which is the term for drill instructor) was there to guide us to scheduled lectures, movies, physical exams, and vaccine injections. He wanted us to look smarter than any other squadron and to sing louder.

One day we were scheduled for a trip to the medics for a huge series of injections—everything from cholera to typhoid. The injections started when we got to Miami Beach and were repeated twice during our stay there, so that by the time we left we were immune to all known and treatable diseases. I stood in line for the first set of four shots (two in each arm) behind a man who was at the very least six feet, six inches. He was so muscular, his muscles had muscles. Holding his shirt in his hand, he advanced to the two medics for his injections. As the first two were given he passed out, going down silently like a Ponderosa Pine. The medics helped him down, gave him his other two shots, and moved him out of the way. Standing up they each took another syringe, looked at me, and said, "Next!" No problem.

In our squadron were many of the Springfield College reservists, and amongst them was a guy named "Zimmy" Zimmerman who was an Olympic level gymnast. When the DI wasn't watching, he would do a front flip and continue marching without missing a beat. This caused a few chuckles, which got the DI's immediate attention. He looked around to find everyone smiling, but Zimmy was looking straight ahead and marching precisely.

My brother Foster had just graduated from Officers Candidate School, and was stationed at Miami Beach in the training program. This was not his idea of what he wanted to do. He was color-blind like me, which meant he could never become a pilot or navigator. He finally left to go to Gunnery School out on the west coast. When he arrived at his new assignment, he wrote me about his trip out there.

On board the civilian train, he met up with a beautiful, inviting (and willing) lady. She was so inviting that when they retired for the evening; he walked down two or three cars in his bathrobe and pajamas to her car and climbed into her berth. During the night, half the train was broken off to go to Los Angeles, including my brother's car with his belongings. The other half went, with my brother blissfully unaware, to San Francisco. What a mess!

Upon arrival there, a red-faced Foster stood on the platform in his bathrobe and pajamas. He looked up and down the platform for an M.P. for help. When he found one, he told his story, and was laughingly supplied with more appropriate clothes and sent on his way to his original destination.

While we were in training at Miami Beach, I wondered where I would end up.

Some lucky bastards were assigned to Aviation Cadet School, which was beyond my reach due to the color-blindness. Both Foster and I had inherited this from our maternal grandfather.

Those new soldiers who had a skill acquired prior to the service were sorted out and kept in that vocation. Naturally, auto mechanics would all go for further training in airplane engine repair. Similarly, those who had an obvious knowledge of radio would be sent to radio school, or radar school. Those of us who had been in college were assigned to the new Army Specialized Training Program, and sent back to college to continue their educations. That included me, and I wondered where I would be sent.

The guys who had been registered as premed students really lucked out. They were shipped to med schools or premed schools to continue their medical education. As for me, I'm damned sure the Air Force didn't give a flying fart about producing Boys' Division secretaries for the YMCA. I hadn't a clue as to where I would end up or what kind of further study I'd be doing. The freshmen and those whose career wishes didn't contribute to the Army needs were a problem.

All of us in that category took loads of tests and were then assigned to a college that the tests indicated would be a good match. In my case, I was less than thrilled to discover that they thought I would be an excellent engineer.

For crying out loud! A bleeping engineer!

All of us "lucky" engineering students left Miami Beach in a troop train for The Citadel in Charleston, South Carolina. This was the reception base where those destined to become engineers gathered from all the other recruit centers. We were about eighteen hundred to two thousand strong.

What a foreboding place this was! In front of the other buildings, there was a huge flag pole, a parade ground, and an assortment of antique cannons. Behind this was the administration building, chow hall, and classroom buildings. To the right of these in a perfect line were the barracks buildings. Each one had thick bars on all the windows, and an equally thick barred gate in the only entranceway. Entering through this gate, I came to a concrete courtyard that was the center of a quadrangle formed by four barracks. From the quadrangle, the center of each barracks had an entrance way to the interior.

It looked like Cheshire Reformatory at home - all stone and bars. Awful!

I gasped when I walked into my assigned room. There was no rug. A bare light bulb hung in the center of the ceiling. There were two tables roughly four feet by three feet in size, sitting on a worn wooden floor. Two straight-backed wooden chairs were at the tables. There was a small study light on each. On one wall there was a piece of furniture referred to as a "Press." At the bottom were four long slots about six inches wide along the entire length. These were for the folded up bed springs and the mattresses each morning.

At each end of the press, there were cubicles for the sheets and blankets, then cubicles for socks and underwear. In the upper center of the press, there was an iron bar extending about five feet to the two rows of cubicles. From this we were instructed to hang class "A" uniforms closest to the cubicles, and fatigues closest to the center.

At reveille, the first thing we did was put the mattresses in the top two slots of the press and then the bed springs in the lower slots, where they were ordered to remain until brought out at taps. This left me either sitting on a stiff chair or standing all day, every day.

We marched to all meals, stood at attention while the commander said grace, and then we sat in unison, maintaining an upright posture, sitting on the edge of the chair, not using the back. All food was eaten at right angles, known in the Army as "eating a square meal." This was the epitome of "Chicken Shit."

When dinner was over, we were called to attention by some officer at the head table, given any necessary orders, dismissed to form outside, and marched to our barracks. After entering the quadrangle, the gate to each quadrangle was closed and locked.

We then studied until 9:00 p.m., when we put the beds up and got in them as taps sounded—not before.

More Chicken Shit.

Thankfully, our stay at this horrible place was short. The Army shipped us out in a week to Georgia Tech. They must have shipped everyone that was at the Citadel in one load. The long troop train rolled right into the station in Atlanta. What an entrance we made!

Georgia Tech was less than three miles from the train station. After loading our duffel bags onto six-by-six trucks, we formed up and marched down Peachtree Street.

Someone in the front of the column started singing "Marching through Georgia," which was picked up by all the troops. We sang just as Sherman's men must have done in the Civil War, singing along and marching smartly. We marched past hundreds of Atlantans and wheeled onto Techwood Drive. We halted in front of our barracks, which were fairly new dorms. Then the order rang out, "Battalion! Halt! Right face!"

We turned ninety degrees to face a four-hundred-foot-long grassy knoll, with the obligatory flag pole, and a group of officers standing there looking at us.

The Commanding Officer stood front and center. His face was beet red. He was furious over our choice of songs. "I won't tolerate this insult to the citizens of Atlanta! Sergeant! Take these songsters on a five-mile tour of the city, and do it at double time, now!"

"Yes sir!" A sergeant with hash marks to his elbow saluted the captain, then wheeled around and glared at us. "Battalion! Attention! Right face! On the double, march!"

We set out on the double for a five-mile-run over some hilly and exhausting streets. The ironic part of having the people of Atlanta along the way cheering and applauding us was not lost on me.

When we returned from our march, we had to find our duffel bags, and then we were assigned rooms in the dorms.

The rooms were suites of two rooms and a bath. In the large room there were two sets of double bunks, and in the smaller room, one set. The dorms had three stories and six entrances per building.

We were assigned to rooms six to a suite and then ordered to pick up our duffels and move into the rooms and await further orders. I have no idea how they assigned us to a room, but the five other guys and I hit it off real well. One fellow was from Idaho, one from South Carolina, one from Illinois, and two from Florida. They were smart and friendly, and the conversation sparkled. As we sat there, Jim from Florida caught a locust about two inches long, or more, in the big room. We were all sitting around talking about it and someone said, "I'll give anyone who eats it two dollars."

The locust was skewered on a big safety pin with its legs moving. Cy Ritchins, the guy from Idaho spoke up, "If all of you put up two dollars, I'll eat it."

"You're on!" came the chorus of replies. CY collected the money and handed it to John to hold, and then put the locust in his mouth, removed the pin and started munching.

"Eew!" "Yuk!" "Gross!" came the cries as we all watched, fascinated. Finally, Cy swallowed.

"How was it?"

"Not bad except the wings got stuck in my teeth." Cy smiled and collected his ten dollars.

Shortly after, we were ordered to fall out for chow, which was down the road, and we were ordered to fall in and marched to the mess hall. The food was good, and the waitresses were even better. The locust was soon a distant memory.

As we settled into the engineering classes, I became more and more convinced that this wasn't for me. I really didn't want to be an engineer. Ironically, if I had stayed in premed at Springfield College, I would have been sent to a premed course somewhere. As it was, I was stuck with a whole pile of physics and mathematics, which I hated.

One Sunday, I decided to go to church, and wound up in of a beautiful church on Peachtree Street. It was huge, and as I approached, the bells were making the air throb, welcoming me to this venerable yellow brick building.

At the beginning of the service, the minister read the announcements, the last of which was, "Mrs. Peyton Wilson cordially invites up to four service men to her home for Sunday dinner. Those interested should wait in the antechamber after the service." That sounded great to me.

After the service I went back to the antechamber to find two other army guys there. None of us knew the other two. I stuck my hand out to each and said, "Hi. I'm Bob Rackliffe."

The nearest guy shook my hand, and then the third guy's hand, saying as he did so, "Hi, Bob, I'm Jim Henderson."

The third guy smiled at us, a big toothy smile, and said, "Howdy. I'm Franklin Powers."

At this point, a black chauffer came up and introduced himself as Thomas, and asked us to please follow him. He had a very pleasant smile and gray hair and was wearing a chauffeur's uniform and holding his chauffeur's hat in his gnarled hand.

When we stepped outside, I was astounded at what I saw.

Right at the front door of the church there was an immaculate car of about vintage 1915. The car was so square it looked as if it were at attention. There were no curves on it anywhere. It was a dull black all over, and the minimal amount of chrome on it looked dull and tired. The windows were at least a quarter inch thick, and had a yellow hue to them.

In the rear sat an elderly lady smiling at us. Jim and I got in the back with Mrs. Wilson, and Franklin sat in the front with Thomas. Mrs. Wilson was wearing a lavender scent that reminded me of Mom. When Thomas started the car, I was thrilled. It was electric! Thomas drove us noiselessly down Peachtree Street, not very far, stopping in front of a yellow brick mansion that had a large porch across the front and around the side. (The bricks were the same color as the bricks on the church.) We three boys got out of the car and turned as a group to help Mrs. Wilson, who was smiling as she extended her hand to Franklin while stepping from the car, and thanked him for his assistance. She was the epitome of Southern graciousness. From the front hall, we entered the sitting room. The walls were a black shiny wood from floor to ceiling. Walking on the thick oriental rugs and the dark parquet floor, we seated ourselves on chairs, which were all heavy dark mahogany. Most had upholstered cushions and backs, but the wooden arms were exposed.

Once seated, Mrs. Wilson turned to Jim and asked, "Now, young man, what is your name, and where is your home?"

"Jim Henderson, ma'am, and I am from Chicago."

"What are you doing now in the army, what do you want to do after the war?"

"I am at Georgia Tech studying to be an engineer, which is great for me, because that is exactly what I wanted to do."

"Well, isn't that wonderful for you. I'm happy for you, Jim." Turning to Franklin, she asked, "And you, young man, what is your name, and what do you want to do after the war?"

"My name is Franklin Powers, ma'am, and I'm from Tennessee. I'm at Georgia Tech also, studying engineering, but I ain't got a hankerin to do that after the war."

"Oh? What would you rather be doing?" Mrs. Wilson asked with a smile.

"My pappy is a pig farmer - biggest one in Mason County," Franklin said proudly, "and I aim on joinin' him."

"Well, I'm sure your father is looking forward to the day when you do join him in the business." Turning towards me, she smiled again and said, "Well, that leaves you young man—tell me all about you."

"My name is Bob Rackliffe, and I'm from Connecticut. I'm at Georgia Tech as well, but like Franklin, I don't have any interest in engineering. I want to study medicine."

Mrs. Wilson nodded and said softly, "It's there for you. All you have to do is aim at it and aim high, because in the long run, you will only achieve that at which you have aimed." She sat quietly for a moment, lost in a sweet memory. "My late husband was a physician."

Jim broke the silence by commenting on the unique car and what fun it was to ride in it. The conversation went on in a lighter vein until Thomas rolled open the pocket doors to the dining room. He was now wearing a butler's uniform with a red and white horizontal striped vest, visible under his butler's coat, and – he was barefoot. "Dinner is served, Mrs. Wilson," he announced.

"Thank you, Thomas," said Mrs. Wilson and then, turning to us, "will you gentlemen join me?"

We followed Mrs. Wilson into the dining room, and I seated her in her chair at the head of the table. I sat at her left facing Jim and Franklin across the table.

The dining room was magnificent, in the same dark color wood as the living room, and along one wall there were floor-to-ceiling windows with attractively brocaded velvet drapes over sheer curtains. The beautifully set table, covered with crystal glasses, crystal plates and gleaming silverware, was itself a masterpiece of carving and exquisite ivory inlay.

There were lace place settings on which double handled soup bowls with a delicious looking soup sat, steam curling up from each bowl. Heavy, brightly polished silverware framed each place setting. Mrs. Wilson said grace and then the meal was served. During the soup course, I watched as Mrs. Wilson noticed that Franklin had not used his napkin sitting to the right of his place setting and had picked up the soup bowl by one of the handles and was drinking the soup. Mrs. Wilson quietly replaced her napkin and raised her bowl to her lips.

Both Jim and I had used our napkins and ate the soup with the soup spoons at our places, but when Mrs. Wilson started drinking the soup holding on to the handles, we quickly followed suit.

The soup was a delicious split pea soup with pieces of ham in it.

"Great soup, Mrs. Wilson!" said Jim.

"Oh, I am happy that you like it. It's an old family recipe."

"This super thick-crusted bread goes great with it," I said.

"Thomas makes the bread. Isn't it wonderful?"

Thomas overheard this and beamed proudly.

The roast beef which Thomas had carved was served with browned new potatoes and a side dish of peas - the best meal since leaving home. Mrs. Wilson kept the conversation going with ease, inquiring about our home lives and parents, until she saw that everyone was through eating. She rang a little bell, which brought Thomas in from the kitchen.

"You may clear now, Thomas."

"Yes'm"

The conversation continued as the dishes were cleared, and when that was accomplished, Thomas brought in crystal finger bowls on lace-covered crystal plates, with each bowl having a flower floating in it. Just as Mrs. Wilson was about to use hers, she saw Franklin remove the flower and drink the water from his bowl. She promptly did the same. Jim and I did not follow on this one. It just looked ridiculous.

For dessert, Thomas brought in a huge silver platter holding homemade peach ice cream. It looked spectacular: a mound of ice cream at least six inches high and twelve inches long - half the size and the shape of an ordinary football. Franklin was served first, and I watched as he removed the empty finger bowl, putting it next to the flower lying on the table. He then helped himself to the ice cream, plopping generous amount of it on his lace covered plate.

I turned to watch Mrs. Wilson, just in time to see her put her lace mat back on the plate before she served herself.

Returning to the university, I pondered Mrs. Wilson's advice which had been softly offered when I said that I wanted to study medicine. "Aim high, because in the long run, you only hit what you aim at."

Meanwhile, the longer I studied the subjects required for an engineering degree, the more I disliked them. When an announcement was made about a need for more pilots, creating openings in the Aviation Cadet program, I saw a way out. I applied, knowing full well that I would have to memorize the Ishihara test for color blindness in order to be accepted.

The Ishihara test was a book full of plates containing circles filled with different color dots that formed numbers or words in them. Some of these numbers or words were visible to the color-blind person, but not to the normal person. Others were completely different numbers and words for the normal person, which the color-blind person could not see.

With the help of a non-color-blind friend, I memorized the right answers in the book from beginning to end, so when I came to the spots that had the word "onion," I would say "color," which was what the non-color-blind person would see. If the number was 27, I would report that there was no number; if I saw "36" I said "83," and so on.

The physical exam was rigorous and thorough.

Not only was every orifice of my body poked and prodded, but a physical fitness assessment was included, which left me sweating and puffing. The eye exam included the Ishihara book, and I waded through like a champion!

Having been accepted as an Aviation Cadet, I was given orders to report for duty at aviation cadet school in Florida after a two week furlough.

I decided to go home.

Luckily, two of my old buddies were home also on their last furloughs before going off to war. It would have been pretty boring to be home alone without having friends home to make it a fun two weeks. The three of us had a pretty fine time together with some of the local girls.

While I was away, my father had purchased chickens, a cow, and a pig named Penelope that was supposedly pregnant. So the old red barn behind the house was once again being used for what it was made for. It was as if Dad had gone back to his childhood days with all these animals to care for, and it did help with all the war time shortages.

He had a high school boy who lived up the street feeding the animals, doing the milking, and collecting the eggs, so that it was not an inconvenience for him. I remember seeing my mother churning milk until she had a lot of butter. Neat!

At the time I came home on furlough, it had become apparent that Penelope was not pregnant. Since Dad had paid for a pregnant pig, he called the farmer who said, "Just ship her back and we'll service her."

When Dad learned that I had two friends home with me, he seized the moment and asked me, "Do you think that you and your two friends could take Penelope back to the farm?" I checked with both of them and they both said, "Sure."

My first thought was to ask John McCabe to help. We were old friends, and since we had been home on leave, he and Irene had double dated with Jane Baldwin - a friend of mine - and me on a couple of occasions.

John was now in the infantry, and he was one big guy, weighing around 220 pounds and all of it muscle. In addition, Don Jones, another old friend of both John and me, was also home from the Marines on his last furlough, too. He was a guy with a "can-do" attitude, and although he wasn't a heavy-weight, he was all muscle, too. Don and I were about the same weight, and I was in pretty good shape, too.

Dad showed us where there was a large supply of oak ceiling molding we could use for the crate sides, after building the frame of the box out of four-by-fours.

Next morning we started, making the floor out of two-by-six inch planks, the corner posts out of 4x4s and the sides out of the 1x4 oak molding, with the entry constructed so that when Penelope was in the crate, the end of the crate could be slid down behind her to bar any exit. The sides were not flush, as there were two to three inches between planks all the way around. It looked foolproof and kept the three of us busy from early morning until about 1:00 p.m.

After a super lunch Mom had made for us, we descended upon Penelope's stall, which was really an old milk room about ten feet by eight. We put the crate just inside the room and directly in front of Penelope, who eyed it in an unsuspecting gaze as we stationed ourselves on each side of her, with John behind her. She was huge! She stood there, chewing something slowly and watching us in a trusting way. At a count of three, Don and I each grabbed an ear, and as John rammed her from behind, we both pulled her by the ears toward the crate. All hell broke loose! First, she kicked with her hind feet, catching John on the chin, and knocking him down in the process. Next she shook both ears loose of Don and me, and growled as she nipped both of us on the hands. She then backed into the corner of the room, glowering at us, pawing the hay, and snorting. She was not going to go peacefully.

The three of us stood there looking at her, attempting to devise another plan of attack.

"We gotta grab her by the legs and shove her as far as we can into the crate, okay?" John said.

On signal, John held her rear legs while Don and I each took a foreleg. At the count of "Three" we all tried to lift her up and push her into the crate. One, two, three Jesus! That pig was galvanized into action in all quarters at the same time. She jerked her right rear leg out and kicked John right in the throat, at the same time nipping Don on the right wrist, and then quickly to the left, where she delivered yet another sharp bite on my wrist.

Falling solidly back to the floor, she snorted, then chased right at John, who was down, gasping for air and holding his throat. Don distracted her by grabbing her tail, whereupon she wheeled like a cougar and clamped her jaws solidly once again on his wrist.

After this victory, Penelope stood in one corner of the stall, pawing the hay while staring balefully at us, alert to any move we might make.

Once again we attacked, holding her muzzle for a short period of time while we tried to put her two front legs in the crate and then push.

This worked until we had her muzzle in as far as we could without having to let go. When that point came, the reversal was quick and calamitous. Penelope was facing out and halfway out of the crate in a heartbeat, daring, just daring, anyone to come near her.

That did it.

After an hour of wrestling, with a lot of sweat and a little blood, I called Dad and gave him the news: the crate was made but we couldn't get Penelope in it.

"I'll send Brian down," said Dad and hung up.

Just like that.

Brian! What on earth was he thinking? Brian had to weigh ninety pounds soaking wet, a sullen sixteen- or seventeen-year-old, and a kid! Surely he was joking!

But he wasn't. About ten minutes later a truck came down the driveway, stopped by the pig stall and out came Mr. Brian. He calmly and silently looked the situation over through his thick lens glasses, without a word except, "Where is your garbage pail?'

"Up on the back porch."

In a minute or two Brian was back at the scene with a bowlful of garbage, which he held under Penelope's nose while leading her into the crate. The back of the crate was slammed home; Brian got back in his truck and left without a word.

The Infantry, Marines, and Air Force looked at each other in disgust. Honor, Duty, Country - and Garbage.

The three of us easily hoisted the crate into the truck and returned Penelope to her old farm, without a word spoken, until John said quietly, "I guess there's more than one way to Philadelphia."

When the furlough was over, I reported to Aviation Cadet School in Florida. The second day there, I was ordered to take a complete physical, which went just fine until I got to the ophthalmologist. Standing in the doorway awaiting my turn, I could see the Ishihara test book had been taken apart, and the pages were out on a counter.

From the doorway (about twelve feet) I could read the test pages the way a normal person could, so when the doctor told me to come in, I said, "I can read them from here, sir."

"No. Come in soldier, and tell me what you see."

That did it. As I walked towards the table, all the bad things appeared, and I could not remember them because they had been removed from the book and reshuffled in a random way.

"Sorry, son, you fail. How did you get this far? Didn't anyone test you?"

"Yes, sir. I memorized the book."

Having failed the flying test, I was ordered to report to Lowery Field in Denver to armament school. The most interesting thing here was learning how to adjust the timing on machine guns for those fighter planes whose guns fired through the propellers. We had to synchronize the firing of the gun with the rotation of the propeller so that the propeller was not hit. This was tricky and fun to do, and you'd better damn well get it right or you were out of armament school!

Other subjects included understanding fuses for bombs and how to set them, machine gun maintenance, etc.

One morning, the commanding officer of the school singled out about twelve men and told us about a new computer-aimed-firing-system that was in the works for a new bomber. He recommended that we go to the school that was being formed for that system. All of us accepted his suggestion and were moved to another part of the base to start learning about the computerized armament system for a new very large bomber called the Super Fortress, or officially, the B-29. This gun-control-system took all the guess work out of where to aim; you didn't have to "lead" the target. All you had to do was circle the fighter in the gun sight, and the computers would move the guns to the correct position to hit the plane.

The 20th USAAF (B-29s) was under the direct command of General of the Armies, Hap Arnold, the Chief of the USAAF. He tolerated no interference from any other general as to how the 20th would be run. The 20th was his baby from the get-go.

In an amazing display of American confidence, before the B-29 had even been built, men were being trained to fly it, learning about its armament, advanced computerized gun turrets, its engines - everything. It was being built for the air war against Japan.

Because this war was being waged by island-hopping, there was need for a bomber with a range far beyond those in service. The B-29 was that plane. It would be capable of three-thousand-mile missions. That it could also carry almost four times the bomb load of a Flying Fortress was an additional huge plus. It had forty stations for five hundred pound bombs in its two bomb bays.

Upon completion of our training in Central Fire Control (as the system was called), I received orders to report to the 377th Bomb Squadron (VH). The letters "VH" stood for Very Heavy and was in reference to the bomb load capacity.

The 377th was stationed in Salina, Kansas, where there were no curves in the roads and no hills. The squadron was part of the 499th Group (VH) which in turn, was attached to the 73rd Wing (VH), of the 20th USAAF. We trained at Salina until the island of Saipan was declared secure.

Saipan was one of the islands in the Marianas chain, which included Guam and Tinian and others, all of which were similar in their beauty and topography. Mt. Tapotchau rose in the center of this irregularly shaped island, on which there were many bays and coves. The water was so clear that what looked six-feet deep was many times deeper, as much as fifty feet.

The Marianas, especially Saipan, which had a garrison of thirty thousand, was the headquarters of the Japanese defense system there. Saipan and Tinian had been in Japanese control for decades. North of the Marianas were the Bonin Islands (which included Pagan and Iwo Jima). These two islands were also heavily fortified by the Japanese. Both of these chains of islands were the chief defensive line for the homeland.

The Marianas were close enough to Japan to serve as bases for the B-29 bombers to be able to bomb the homeland and return to them without refueling.

Since Saipan was headquarters in the Marianas chain of islands, the defenses on that island were everywhere and thorough. Because of the ominous defenses there, being attacked by the Americans in June of 1944 was a complete surprise. By the first night, the 2nd and 4th Marine divisions and the 27th Army division were all on land, with a beach head of several hundred yards. The night was full of savage counter-attacks by the Japanese Army, which consisted of thirty thousand men on the twelve-by-five mile island. The terrain was hilly and full of coral caves. All the native (Chamorro) people had been so brainwashed that they believed the Americans would kill them and rape them. Many of them, when cornered, committed suicide by jumping off cliffs with their children in their arms to the water three hundred feet below.

The numerous caves in the soil-covered-coral were an especially unique problem. The Japanese darted in and out of them, or rolled out their artillery, firing, then rolled them back into the safety of the caves. Marines solved this problem by using flame throwers on them, as they joked, "If they don't come out, it will be their ashes."

During the battle for the island, the army division's commanding general was replaced by Army General Holland ("Howling Mad") Smith to more adequately match the fighting ability of the Marines. The island was declared secure in three days with five thousand of the defending army still alive and scattered about the island, hiding in caves. The Japanese commanding general and his staff officers committed hari-kari.

The cost of this battle was twenty-five thousand Japanese, fourteen thousand Americans, and an unknown number of Chamorros.

In addition to the victory on land, the invasion brought forth the majority of the Japanese Naval Air Force, and resulted in their overwhelming defeat in what became known as the "Great Marianas Turkey Shoot."

There was an intense naval battle raging at the same time, which became known as the "Battle of Philippine Sea." It was the greatest sea battle ever fought. The Japanese lost two carriers and six hundred planes.

For all intents and purposes (except in homeland defense), their Japanese naval air force was reduced to nuisance raids, and their navy retired towards the home land. They were low on fuel and, due to the destruction of their merchant fleet by U.S. submarines; there was little hope for them that this shortage would be corrected.

As soon as Saipan was declared secure, the building of Isley Field on the northern end of the island started. It consisted of two landing strips of sufficient length to accommodate the huge aircraft that would be using it. The runways had to be lengthened considerably to allow the heavy laden huge planes room for take off and landing. Surrounding the perimeter of the two runways had parking places for all the planes, all in a row.

In November of 1944, the 73rd Bomb Wing took off for Saipan in the Marianas, and the ground crews, of which I was a part, were flown there by Military Air Transport, aka MATS. The ground crews were shipped to San Francisco by troop train, which took us three days to get from Kansas to San Francisco. Troop trains had no priority, so that if the track had to be cleared for oncoming traffic, troop trains gave way. We finally arrived at the station in San Francisco and were transported to our barracks in six-by-six trucks. On the way, we saw the beautiful Golden Gate Bridge and Alcatraz out in the bay. We were in San Francisco for just a couple of days.

We left for Hawaii on the day after all four of my wisdom teeth were extracted. As we flew west, I remember looking at the Golden Gate Bridge and wondering if I'd ever see it again.

Our destination in Hawaii was Hickam Field on Oahu, but landing there required three attempts by our pilot due to the violent updrafts once the plane was over land. The aborted attempts all came while we were over the extinct volcano at Diamond Head. Looking down into the volcano, all I could see in the crater was grass.

When we landed, we were greeted by USO ladies offering us cups of pineapple juice that tasted so good, I thought it was fresh. It was so good that when I got in to the barracks I announced, "Hey, guys! The USO ladies are giving out fresh pineapple juice! You have to try it!"

A pile of guys went down to try it, and when they came back, they were all over me for giving them bad info. Their juice came out of Dole pineapple cans, which were cut open on their arrival.

The next day we flew to Midway, where we refueled. How desolate! You could see one end of the island from the other, and there was nothing but a few palm trees and sand around the air strip. The only thing that made the heat bearable was the constant breeze.

Next stop was Kwajalein for refueling. A radio repairman came on board, and I was surprised to see a friend from my home town, George Abraham.

"Hey, Abba! How're you doing? You stationed here?"

"Hi, Bob! I'm doing okay. What's up with you? Where're you heading?"

"Saipan," I replied. "What do you hear about it, George?"

"It's plenty hot there right now," he replied (and he wasn't talking about the weather). "They've declared that island secure with five thousand Japs still running around loose."

That information reinforced the feeling of fear in me.

We stopped one more time for fuel at Eniwetok, and took off for our final destination immediately after refueling.

The 73rd Bomb Wing (VH) received a welcome to Saipan from "Tokyo Rose" the day they landed there. Not only did she name the numbers of the wing, groups, and squadrons, she named the commanders of each unit, right down to the squadrons. She reassured us that we were all going to be annihilated by the Imperial Japanese Army and Air Force. I wondered how she got so many details right.

On the very first night on Saipan, I was put on guard duty in a bomb dump, which was in front of and below the extended airstrip. Around the bombs there was vegetation that looked like sugar cane. I was scared to death and felt surrounded by the five thousand Japanese still on the island, whose main objective was to kill Bob Rackliffe.

Holding my carbine with the safety off and listening to every sound, I heard some noises in the cane, and I shouted, "Halt! Who goes there?" three times as required. Receiving no answer, I emptied my carbine in the direction of the noise. This brought the Sergeant of the Guard and others rapidly to the scene. A search of the area with guns poised led us to a very dead pig.

The 73rd Wing was the first wing of the 21st Bomber Command of the 20th Air Force to see action over Japan from the Marianas. There had been six bombings by the B-29s of the 20th Bomber Command based in India and China against the Japanese homeland. In their first raid, sixty-three planes took part with poor results, and they lost seven planes and fifty-five men. From then on they limited their targets to Manchuria. The 20th Bomber Command was under the direction of General Curtis LeMay, who had been the commander of the eighth Air Force in Europe but had been ordered by General Arnold to the Pacific in April 1944 to take over the Pacific bombing campaign.

The B-29s in China and India were eventually moved to the Marianas. General LeMay was relieved of command of the Twentieth, and ordered to take command of the twenty first[t] Bomber command in January 1945. He set up his headquarters at Guam.

From the Marianas, each bombing mission was a three thousand mile round trip. The planes were under attack for fifteen hundred miles (from Iwo Jima to Japan, and back to Iwo Jima).

The Japanese fighters would come up from Iwo Jima when their radar indicated our presence or when they were warned by radio from their troops on Pagan Island, which was between us and Iwo Jima. They would attack all the way to Japan. At that point, with their fuel exhausted, they would be replaced by new fighters taking off from the homeland to attack us all the way back to Iwo Jima, where they would break off the engagement and land at Iwo Jima to await the next attack.

In our squadron, eighteen of our original twenty flight crews were lost on these long missions. Some were shot down by anti-aircraft fire, others by fighter planes, and still others by damage that occurred while under attack, making the return flight impossibly long. Others, low on fuel, started dumping anything detachable out the hatches to lighten the load in an attempt to reach home. All along the planned flight route, the Navy had ships and subs posted to pick up survivors from planes that ditched due to enemy action. The Navy succeeded in saving countless numbers of downed crewmen.

When the time came for the planes' return from a raid, all the ground crew would assemble on the airfield (which was referred to as the "line") and wait for their planes to appear.

The first planes would be seen turning on their landing lights, one after another as they came in to touch down finally on safe ground. Red flares came shooting out of many of them, signifying there were wounded aboard. Landings were unpredictable and gut-wrenching.

Planes with only two or three engines running ("dead" engines having their props "feathered" and therefore useless) were just making the airstrip, while others with parts of wings and rudder missing were staggering in, just dropping and skidding sideways to a stop. Still others landed on their bellies due to landing gear damage, screeching in metal-rending slides into other planes off the runway altogether. Many planes had bullet holes, shrapnel tears, and parts of wings, rudders, and fuselages missing or damaged.

This was the scene after our first foray onto the Japanese homeland, which was textbook and a failure in every way. First: we flew in and bombed from 30,000 feet with our superior bombsights. This altitude demanded more gasoline, so one bomb bay was carrying reserve gasoline tanks instead of bombs.

Second: the effect of the wind from that altitude had not been considered, and the result was that most bombs were blown by the wind off their intended targets, and most landed in the sea.

Third: The computerized gunsights were not aimed properly and were essentially useless. After that first raid, every bomber was taken out to a station between the two runways, and the gun sights and the guns were aimed at the distant top of Mt. Tapotchau. This meant that every gun on the plane and every gunsight were aiming at the same point. From then on, the input to the computers aimed the guns at the right place to hit the target. All that was needed was for the gunner to keep the attacking plane circled in his gun sight, and the computers would aim the guns at the right place to score. It was a deadly system when set up properly.

Additionally, on that first raid, the Japanese learned quickly that in a head-on attack, the computers were too slow and were firing behind them as they approached.

This computer error was immediately corrected before the next mission.

The war wasn't going just one way though, and the Japanese retaliated immediately. Because of their limited range, they would fly their planes down to Iwo Jima at night, and then to Pagan Island the next night, keeping them camouflaged during the day. In this manner, they brought down Betty bombers and Zero (Zeke) fighters, so when our planes were returning from a mission to the Japanese homeland, the Betties joined in with the returning planes, turning on their landing lights until over our field, at which time they shut them off, and dropped their bombs, and escaped into the night.

Another night, a Betty arrived and bombed the airfield successfully. It was then caught in the anti-aircraft lights as it attempted to flee, while all our anti-aircraft guns were firing at it.

It was a clear night, and in a deadly way, it was beautiful to see the silver plane like a moth at a street light, trying to evade the gunfire, which was bursting all around it.

It did so successfully, only to encounter our P-61 night fighters (known as Black Widows, due to their all black exterior and deadly computerized firing system), which brought it down with two or three deadly bursts of its four fifty-caliber machine guns and twenty-millimeter cannon.

The entire 73rd bomb wing was housed at the northernmost part of the island on a ledge that bordered the ocean. It was about 150–200 feet below the airfield. Each squadron was constructed the same way: a mess hall, which was central, and an area near it that had four speakers for a P.A. system atop a telephone pole. At the base of the pole was a rack designed to hold helmets, plus some unbreakable mirrors, and fifty-gallon drums of water for shaving and washing.

The officers' quarters and their club were separate from the enlisted men, and closer to the ocean. The administration building was adjacent to the mess hall on the east side. On the west side were the enlisted men's tents and gang shower. All the ground crews were living in eight-man pyramidal tents with the sides rolled up. Next to each cot, each man had made a foxhole and surrounded it with sandbags, for use in the event that we were attacked.

And we were. It was noon, and we were all down from the airfield for lunch. The P.A. speakers were playing the music from *Oklahoma* when suddenly, from the east end of our encampment, a brilliant green Japanese Zero ("Zeke") fighter with huge orange "meatballs" came roaring at us with guns blazing.

He was no more than one hundred fifty feet above the camp. Reaching the other end of the line of tents, he did a tight turn and started back towards us. Again the guns were flashing as he swept over us. Almost at the end of the run east of us, our anti-aircraft got him. He wheeled left and nose up, exploded and crashed right in the middle of the 500th bomb group.

It was terrifying, and yet beautiful. All the while, from the four speakers on the telephone pole, the music from *Oklahoma* was playing the song that started, "Out of a dream." It was bizarre. During all the shooting, noise, and confusion, that song kept playing, and I kept thinking of Jane in that red velvet evening gown with the white net skirt, dancing to the music, as she had done at a sorority dance we had attended. Despite the roar of anti-aircraft guns and the rat-a-tat-tat of the machine guns, it was as if nothing was happening except Jane was dancing.

I was captivated.

An attack also occurred in broad daylight as the ground crews were working on the planes, this one by a single "Zeke" who came in strafing the planes that were all lined up in straight rows (something I never understood).

At the outset of that attack, I was working on the upper gun turret about fifteen to twenty feet above the ground. When that plane came over, and I heard the bullets whining off the tarmac, I was off that plane and high-tailing for safety in one single move. Looking back, I could see that only a fool would make a jump like that.

Hello, fool.

While we were bombed and strafed a few times, the ground crews were not really in any danger from the large contingent of Japanese soldiers, still on the island and at large. However, they had the full attention of the Marines. At our first assembly in our new quarters, our commanding officer transmitted an order from the island commanding general: "Air Force personnel will not engage the enemy, should that unlikely event occur. That is the responsibility of the Marines."

That was fine with me, thank you very much.

One Sunday, when we were quiet, my friend George Radford and I were walking along a dirt path, looking for some bananas (which were small but plentiful there).

George asked me, "Bob, what are you going to do after the war? Got any plans or ideas?"

"Gosh, I've given that a lot of thought. I feel like I was put here for a reason, and I think I know where that is coming from. How about you?"

"I feel the same way. It just doesn't seem right that we are supposed to worry about ourselves, and not be concerned about other people who might be in trouble. I have talked this over with my fiancée, Rita, and I think I would like to try to become a veterinarian. That would put me where I could help a lot of people."

"You know, I think you and I are on the same wavelength. We are meant to help others. I think I would like to go back and give medicine another try. I really wasn't educated or dedicated enough the first time I tried. I'm sure I could do better, and I can't imagine a field more satisfying. I feel the hand of God in what has happened to me so far. As a doctor, I could be of service to God by serving my fellow man."

"That's exactly the way I feel too, Bob. Let's shake hands on that and pledge to each other that we will dedicate ourselves to his service."

A firm warm handshake affirmed the pledge.

We stood there on that dirt road, overlooking Saipan's Magicienne Bay, and shook hands pledging ourselves to this worthwhile task. I felt as if my future had just been pointed out to me, and I'm sure George did, too.

It was good feeling.

We had just turned a corner after greeting a marine squad out on patrol, when some shots rang out and we heard bullets whiz by. The marines heard the shots, too, because they came back into view on the double and spotted a Japanese soldier climbing up a cliff on the other side of a bay, about four hundred feet away. He was heading for a cave, and the marines let him get there. As he rose up to walk in, they opened fire and watched him fall about forty feet into the water.

George and I became very close friends. He was from Atlanta. His interest in becoming a veterinarian and my determination to go back to medicine were just another example of the many things we had in common, such as our family life at home, especially classical music and involvement in our churches, and generally we just formed a true friendship, enjoying being together. We were both fed up with the ever-present discussions of sexual postwar plans that were constantly the subject of conversation by many of the troops. That discussion was endless, and pointless, considering our circumstances. Oh, I'm sure we both had our carnal moments, but the main task was to get home again. We had no lack of things to talk about, and enjoyed our time together.

From November 1944 to December 1944, the bombing continued during the day time from high altitude, with results that did not please General LeMay. (He questioned whether we needed to fly at such altitudes.) Our targets were against their industry. The Mitsubishi engine plant in Nagoya, oil storage depots, ball bearing factories, etc. We were using five hundred pound bombs, twenty per plane, in raids that grew to two hundred or more bombers.

It was clear though, that the island of Iwo Jima had to be taken, in order to eliminate the damage and loss of life it caused while it was in Japanese hands. From late November to the end of the year, Japanese forces caused havoc with scores of Betty bombers and fighters damaging or destroying more than forty aircraft of ours.

On February 19, 1945, with great heroism and staggering losses, the marines secured the last thorn in the side of the air force, and in the following days raised the flag on Mt. Suribachi as they continued the fierce battle to victory. Finally, the island was declared secure, allowing damaged planes to land there when making it to Saipan was impossible due to damage.

The crew of the first plane that landed there was killed by Japanese who slit open their tents in the middle of the night and stabbed them to death.

This left the Japanese air force at Pagan Island cut off from their homeland. They were starving to death, as no Japanese boats had come to them. Consequently, our P-51 fighter escorts started dropping K rations to them from their wing racks. After the garrison got used to running onto the airfield to get the rations, the P-51s armed their wing racks with antipersonnel bombs for one last flight.

Following the example of the British in Europe and using the single plane formation devised by General LeMay, huge changes in our bombing strategy were made. All the guns were removed from the planes as were the bomb bay tanks (thus allowing each plane to double bomb capacity). Removing all of this equipment and doubling the bomb load required that we lower our altitude to between 5,000 and 8,000 feet to ensure that there would be sufficient gasoline for the round trip. The planes were all painted black on their bottom surfaces, and the change to nighttime bombing was ordered.

General LeMay also ordered a change to fire bombing, as most Japanese buildings were flammable. On February 4, 1945, the first fire bombing raid took off from Saipan, with each plane carrying napalm and or phosphorous bombs in clusters of six bombs per station. That was a total of two hundred forty firebombs per plane. They flew into Tokyo at 5,000 feet with General LeMay in the lead plane and the others following in a line without a formation. Directly after the bombs were released and hit the ground, they exploded, showering flaming napalm in all directions, starting fires everywhere. The Japanese fire department came out and extinguished many fires after the raid, but after that, and for the duration of the fire raids, there were five incendiary bombs and one delayed fuse anti-personnel bomb per station on each aircraft.

That took care of the fire department.

Then we started burning Tokyo. On the first Tokyo mission, there were two hundred eighty-five bombers that dropped two thousand tons of incendiaries on the city, being careful to avoid -on government orders - the Imperial Palace. The resulting blaze caused a firestorm, which raised the temperature to thousands of degrees, causing objects (including humans) to burn spontaneously, and accounted for over 80,000 deaths, thousands of injured and burned bodies, and over a million homeless.

In that one raid, seventeen square miles of Tokyo were burned to the ground.

All the larger cities in Japan, and fifty to sixty smaller ones, suffered the same fate starting from that fateful night.

From the start of the fire raids on, days melted into weeks, and the havoc continued until the invasion of Okinawa, which started on March 26, 1945.

A huge part of the U.S. Navy was involved on that massive invasion of an island always considered Japanese. The preparations to defend the island had been ongoing for years. There were many caves from which large cannon could be rolled out, fired, and then rolled back in. The battle was the biggest of the Pacific war, both on the ground and at sea, where the British Navy (which included units of the Australian and Canadian

Navies) and the American Navy assembled more than forty-five carriers, thirteen battleships and a total of thirteen hundred naval vessels in all.

The Japanese fleet sailed out of harbor at Kobe with the battleship Yamato in the lead, intent on fighting through the allied Navy, and ultimately planning to beach itself on the shore of Okinawa, whereupon it would turn its cannon on the attackers. It was sunk on April 7th before the plan could be achieved.

The Japanese response to the attack on Okinawa was to start sending Kamikaze (Divine Wind) planes at the fleet. These were suicide missions where the pilot of the plane was intent on crashing his plane into a warship; the bigger the better. The Kamikaze attacks involved fifteen hundred Japanese planes and sank twenty ships, as well as damaging at least twenty-five others. The impact on the Navy was so severe that the entire Twentieth Air Force (us) was taken off of our job of bombing industrial targets and towns and assigned the task of making take off from any airport in the homeland impossible by destroying their airfields and air strips. To achieve this aim, we switched from carrying incendiaries to forty-five hundred pound bombs per plane, and with flights of one hundred fifty to three hundred fifty planes per attack. Thus armed, we sought out enemy airfields and strips, also gasoline supplies near the fields, which were blown apart, making them totally inoperable.

While doing this in March and early April, we were flying right over Kobe, Japan, where the entire Japanese fleet lay at anchor before it went to sea. We had strict orders not to bomb it, as it was a "Navy Target."

Think of it: two hundred fifty bombers, each with forty-five hundred pound bombs, and the attack was left to Navy dive bombers, which had a maximum load of four five hundred pound bombs per plane. I lost a high school friend in one of those Navy bombers, who cart wheeled to his death while attacking that fleet.

Some time in June there was a story going around that a new group of B-29s had landed on Tinian (which you could see from Saipan), and they were pretty isolated, but told everyone that they were going to end the war.

And they did.

On August 6th the Enola Gay with Colonel Paul Tibbets in command took off from Tinian, and headed north with two other B-29s. When they got to Hiroshima, the bomb bay doors opened and "Little Boy" was let loose to convince the Japanese to surrender. It exploded in the air above the city, killing ninety thousand in the first minute, but ultimately killed one hundred forty thousand when the deaths from radiation were added. Despite this attack, Japan refused to surrender.

On August 9th, Nagasaki was atomic-bombed, killing eighty thousand. The same day, the Russians - who had been asked by the Japanese in April to broker a peace with the Allies - invaded Manchuria. Stalin never mentioned the request of the Japanese to the allies, wanting to see the effects of the atomic bomb, on which he was briefed at Yalta. He used the knowledge to time his grab of Manchuria on the day the bomb was dropped. On that day, Russian troops crossed the border of Manchuria, and it has been in their hands ever since.

Japan surrendered on the 15th of August, unconditionally.

Everyone was given a double ration of beer to celebrate, and the cooks did themselves proud the day the surrender was announced, but by nightfall, we were all on the line addressing the immediate priority for our

Command, which was to get supplies in to the prison camps as soon as possible. It was estimated that it would be at least a week before the Navy could get ashore and get to the prison camps, so we were the first positive sign of hope that the prisoners would see.

We welded oil drums together, joining their ends, then filled them with medicines, clothes, food, candy, shoes, bandages, toilet articles, toilet paper—anything we thought they could use. The ends of the drums were then shut with a wooden circle, held in by a piece of two-by-four that was kept in place by large nails driven through the oil drum, deeply into ends of the two-by-fours.

Depending on the weight of the welded drums, three or four brightly colored yellow or red parachutes were attached to the drums, and the drums were then suspended from a bomb station. For three days and nights, no one slept as we labored to get the help up to the prisoners.

As the flights of mercy continued, many of the ground crew was invited to make the trip up and see the camps, the country, and also to fly over Hiroshima. I jumped at the opportunity to see all this that had been such a huge part of my life for so long.

Even the takeoff was exciting. I had seen hundreds of planes dive out of sight at the end of the runway, and I knew it was in order to gain speed for the ascent, but sitting in the ring gunners chair and watching the sea come right up at us was damned scary!

After a few hours, we passed over Iwo Jima, which did look like a pork chop, and I couldn't help but think of all the guys who had lost their lives there, for the sake of the air war against Japan.

When we arrived at the prison camp, we came in low, and there were a tremendous number of smiles and waving from the thin occupants of the camp. We waggled those huge wings, then climbed up to an altitude that would give the chutes time to open, and sent them swaying on their way in a colorful display.

The prisoners were all waving and smiling as we "bombed" them with the oil drums. Most landed safely and nearby, but one failed to open all the chutes, and fell into the camp striking a group of men.

It was a sad thought that maybe we had killed someone—maybe even someone who had made it this far after surviving the "Death March from Bataan."

After we had dropped our supplies and waggled our wings over the camp again as a promising sign that more would be coming, we headed toward Hiroshima, which was in the western part of the island of Honshu. One of the reasons it was picked as the target was that there were no prisoner of war camps there.

What devastation! Roads were visible, with the rest being ash, an occasional girder still stood upright, but there was nothing left standing for as far as I could see. We were down to about five hundred feet, and I was looking out an open hatch at an old woman who was wearing a straw coolie hat. She looked up at us and waved tentatively. How pathetic.

With the end of the war, the huge Army of the United States started to disband—an event planned for by the Chiefs of Staff. It went smoothly, too, and was based on a point system; e.g., one point for every month in service, points for combat time, and points for battles, etc. The more points one had, the quicker one would be sent home and discharged. At the time I had fifty-three points, and they were discharging men who had ninety-plus.

Females could be discharged, just by requesting discharge from their superior officer.

I figured I'd be around a long time on Saipan. So we had time to spare after cleaning up all that we could at the base. All the air crews were gone in the first two weeks, and the officers' barracks were empty and silent.

One day, George and I managed to have the use of a jeep, so we took off for the opposite end of the island to see the airstrip that had been used by fighter planes of the Navy. It was a very small strip, laid down between two cliffs that were at least three hundred feet above the unbelievably clear water of Magicienne Bay. When we arrived there, we watched in amazement as one after another F6Fs and F4U fighter planes were pushed over the cliff by bulldozers.

These were not junk planes, but operational. They were simply not needed any more. It was sad to see those magnificent planes just thrown away.

Watching one F4U going on its last flight reminded me of one day when a trio of Marine F4Us with their gull wings had come in to Isely field in formation, buzzed the field, then all three pulled up into a tight loop, lowered their wheels and landed all in one motion and in perfect formation.The loop couldn't have been more than forty-five feet from the ground.

Hot Dogs and marvelous to watch, as those who saw cheered their acrobatics.

PART 3:

HOMECOMING

B y November, the required point count to be discharged was down to sixty-five, so when I was summoned to the first sergeant's desk and told to pack up because I was listed for departure to the states on the next ship, I was dumbfounded. Then I realized that they were counting my months in the Reserve, which was wrong. I asked to speak with the captain (who, I'm sure had had his fill of guys complaining that their points were wrong).

He made short shrift of me after I told him I thought there was a mistake in my point count. I'm sure that the poor man had heard nothing but the "mistakes" in point counts ever since the war had ended

"Damn it, sergeant! You are an enlisted man! You are not supposed to think! Now get the hell out of here!"

I saluted and said, "Yes, sir!"

Two days later about forty of us were loaded onto six-by-sixes, and taken to the harbor where we offloaded on a dock next to a huge gray ship. It was an attack troop transport, and in six-foot letters on the side were the letters APA237. It also had a name: Fort Lauderdale. At two or three gangplanks leading into the ship, there were masses of soldiers waiting to board. My squadron members and other squadrons from our group were at the forward one, which led us in to the bow of the boat. When ordered, we went aboard and down a stairway, which was dammed close to being a ladder, into the bow section of the ship. This was one big room filled with paired bunks, separated by an aisle of about three feet from more paired bunks. The whole area was just paired bunks and aisles filling the space, and of course, decreasing in width to accommodate the shape of the bow. The bunks were stacked five bunks high to the ceiling. Resting your elbow on the frame of one bunk, you could touch the bunk above with your finger tips.

At about noontime on that bright and sunny day, the ship started out of the harbor of Saipan smoothly. As I watched the island falling astern, I felt a feeling of joy and hope for the future. An indescribable feeling of relief that I had made it was coupled with sorrow for the guys who hadn't.

No sooner had we left the harbor at Saipan on this eleven-day journey back to the States, when we felt the boat start to rise and fall on the waves, which were about six to eight feet. It didn't take much time before evidence of sea sickness began to appear. Red Smith, a bow-legged Texan from our outfit, was standing next to me at the rail watching the departure, got a real desperate look on his face, and promptly threw up over the rail. He turned green and left for the bow bunkroom. I did not see him again for at least five days. It was pretty obvious that the seasick guys, of whom there were many, would sleep in the lower bunks. The only troublesome part of this arrangement was that the floor tended to be a bit tricky to walk on.

Fortunately for me, I was not in the least bit seasick, and got a kick out of going up and down the stairs, because if you timed it right with the waves, you could go up or down weightlessly. This was going to take eleven days to get to San Diego, and I noticed on the first day that they were grabbing guys to do KP and to clean the bunk rooms (ugh!), so I made up my mind to stay out of sight. For the entire trip I avoided any work parties and I spent my time outside the cable guard rails that lined the deck and on the sea side of lifeboats that were all along the perimeter of the deck outside the guard rail.

No one could see me there, and since we had beautiful weather the entire trip I was able to stay, unseen, every day. I read and watched the ocean and saw my first flying fish.

Going to the bathroom was an interesting and exciting experience. There was a trough about thirty feet long with pairs of slats placed in an anatomically correct position over two thirds of the trough. The remaining third was for voiding. Salt water came surging up from the sea via a four inch pipe at one end of the trough, and exited at the other end at a constant and rapid rate back to the sea again.

Not a day went by that did not have a hot seat party. With five or more guys doing their business, some one would bunch up a huge wad of toilet paper, light it and set it adrift downstream. This was a constant source of amusement, as well as a warning to be alert.

Mess was another experience common to Navy guys I guess, but very different for land lubbers. We ate standing, not sitting, around tables, five to a side. Frequently, as the ship rolled to its side in twenty-foot waves, dishes would slide away from the person whose food it was, only to come back when the ship rolled the other way. This was happening frequently on the day poor Red Smith staggered down for his first food in a week. He stood at the table and ate his whole bowl of oatmeal. Just as he finished it the bowl slid away from him as the table slanted. Shortly it returned to his place, full of someone else's vomit. Red sort of half moaned and half screamed and leapt up the ladder as if he'd been shot from a gun. I never saw him again.

As we got to within two days of home, the anticipation was palpable. I could hardly wait to sail up under the Golden Gate Bridge with people lining it to cheer us home as we came into the harbor at San Francisco.

Except we didn't go to San Francisco, we didn't go under any bridge, there was no band playing when we docked in San Diego, and there were no people cheering.

Nothing. While we all felt like heroes, the heroes had come home in August, and this was November.

Nobody working at the dock gave a damn. We were just human cargo being shipped to the States via San Diego, which had had enough of servicemen and their needs already. The city was in a "let's get back to living the way we did before the war" mode.

"Okay, soldiers grab your duffels and disembark. Line up on the dock as soon as you reach your group." When our group was all off the ship, we were then loaded on six-by-sixes and driven off to a barracks somewhere on the outskirts of the city. We went into a standard army mess hall, with the kitchen at one end behind the tables of food. On the other side of this food serving station were rails guiding the troops through as they picked out their food. The meal that was being served that night was predictably lousy. It was more mutton (from New

Zealand, I suppose). I'm sure the "Kiwis" must have killed every dammed goat or old ewe and dumped them on the U.S. at ridiculous prices. It seemed to me that I had been living on mutton for a year.

The next move was to get each man's discharge destination on paper, and passes for the railroad to take him to that place. It was done without a hitch in less than an hour, which surprised the hell out of me. We had two weeks to report to our discharge station. Mine was Camp Devens, where I had started my army experience two years earlier. Soldiers were going in all directions from here to the places where they would be discharged; usually back to the station where they had been inducted.

At mess that first night, I sat next to an Air Force sergeant who was leaving the next day. His name was Nate, and he was heading east for Atlanta. He told me about flying home. "You know if you want to go home by air, all you have to do is show up with your duffel at MATS (Military Air Transport Service) at the airport and sign in. They'll get you home, maybe not in a straight line, but it sure as shit beats those fucking trains."

Well! That sounded pretty dammed fine to me, recollecting my train ride from Kansas to San Francisco taking seven days (troop trains had no priority and spent many many hours on sidings).

"Mind if I join you, Nate?"

"Hell, no, Bob. I'd appreciate the company." We left the mess hall and strolled around that God-forsaken place, smoking a couple of Lucky Strikes. We agreed to meet outside the mess hall at six o'clock the next morning and have breakfast together.

Next morning at six o'clock I saw Nate coming towards me with a big grin on his handsome face. His dark eyes sparkled, and he had a pair of dimples framing a perfect set of white teeth. "Hey there, Bob! Sleep okay? This is our day, Bobby boy, this is our day!"

I don't know which of us was more excited. Even the breakfast of one apple, coffee, and the creamed chip beef on toast (known as "Shit on a Shingle" in army parlance) did not dampen the mood. Actually, though I would never admit it to anyone, I liked SOS.

After breakfast Nate said, "Let's go down to Motor Transport and see if we can hitch a ride to the airfield."

"Good idea," I replied, "if that doesn't pan out we can always grab a taxi." There were scads of taxis hanging around this base, because most everyone there was going somewhere else.

A couple of pilots were getting into a jeep right outside the entrance to the Motor Transport unit.

Nate called out, "Lieutenant! Are you heading for the airport?"

"I sure am, sergeant. You boys need a lift?"

"Yes sir!" We answered in a chorus.

"Throw your duffels in and climb aboard. We're almost ready for takeoff."

And take off we did. There were many times in that ride when it was a three-wheeled jeep, but we arrived at MATS intact. Everyone had a cigarette going as soon as we stopped and unloaded.

Nate and I hopped over the side, grabbed our duffels, and headed for the waiting room. One of the lieutenants followed us in with his B-4 bag after saying good bye to his friend, and we all went up to the desk to sign in.

The soldier behind the counter took care of the lieutenant first, getting him on a plane to Chicago, and then turned to us.

"Now, what about you guys?" The soldier looked at us and added, "Everything east of Knoxville is shut down due to weather. Where are you heading?"

"Atlanta," said Nate.

"Bradley or Westover," I said.

"Too bad. I can only get you as far as Knoxville right now, but you know by the time you get there the weather may have broken up in the East."

"Well, it sure is closer to New England than this is. I'll go," I said.

"So will I," said Nate.

We grabbed our bags and headed out to the plane that was being serviced. An officer was walking around the plane inspecting the wings, rudder, and undercarriage. He looked at us and smiled. "Hi guys! Heading east?"

"Yes sir."

"Well, climb aboard this old crate, and make yourself comfortable if you can. We'll be leaving in about ten minutes. Have you eaten?"

"No sir." Well, it had been two-plus hours since breakfast.

"Well go back to the USO counter and get a couple of sandwiches and some coffee. You might even get a couple extra for the trip. They are home made and dammed good!" Looking at his watch he added, "You have plenty of time."

Those ladies from the USO gave us delicious roast beef sandwiches, chocolate chip cookies and coffee that was really coffee. When we left, they provided us with a little stash of sandwiches and cookies for the trip.

At the time of takeoff, Nate and I were the only passengers along with a few boxes. This C-47 (a civilian DC3) had long, one-piece aluminum benches with indented seats and backs. The benches ran the length of the plane and faced each other. There were no windows. The seats had belts, but no cushions. Since Nate and I were the only passengers, we could spread our overcoats over the seat indentations and lie down on them to sleep. This was slightly uncomfortable, but our overcoats helped make it feel pretty good.

At take off, Nate and I sat upright and strapped ourselves in. The plane's engines roared as the plane rattled down the runway and into the air, slowly climbing to our assigned altitude. It was a bumpy ride, as there was a lot of rough weather around us. On occasion, the pilot would request and receive permission to change altitude. All in all, the ride to Knoxville was conducive to sleeping and eating the rest of those delicious sandwiches.

We landed and taxied up to the terminal in Knoxville. When the plane stopped, we unbuckled, thanked the pilot for the really fine ride, and headed in to the terminal to see what would be our next move.

The weather up to Newark and the rest of the eastern U.S. was so bad that most of the pilots, including Nate's, were electing to wait in Knoxville. All, that is, except one stud that came out to the waiting area and announced, "I've got a date in New York City tonight, and even though the weather is crappy, I'm going. Does anyone want to go to Newark with me?"

Old stupid me, put my hand up. *only me?* I thought. *What the hell am I in for now?*

Terror—that's what.

I said good bye to Nate, who tried to talk me out of going, "It's too bad up that way, Bob. Wait here—there will be other flights." But I had said I'd go, so I winked at Nate and said, "Nah, everything will be fine, Nate.

You have a good trip home, and I'm sure glad we got together."

As I headed out to the plane, I noticed the pilot did not do the usual on-ground inspection. The two of us boarded the plane. I was his only passenger.

The engines sputtered into action. We trundled down towards the runway with its fog shrouded blue lights, wheeled onto it, and waited for clearance. Once that was given, the engines roared into full throttle, and we gathered speed as we hurtled down the runway, soon lifting off, feeling the thump of the wheels coming up.

We crossed over the Alleghenies; at least that's what the pilot told me. I couldn't see them, but I could sure feel them. From the moment we were airborne, we hit severe turbulence that kept dropping the plane. Each time we hit a down draft, I thought the wings would get torn off, then they would find some air under us and we would start to climb back up, with the engines straining to regain the altitude. My entire body was in the air on the first drop. I quickly buckled myself in. The hair-raising drops and the Pratt and Whitney engines were locked in a battle over which force would win, but over a period of three or four hours the old "war horse" of the Army Air Force again proved its reliability. It was without a doubt the worst experience I have ever had in an airplane, but I was grateful that if I had to go through it, I was in a C-47.

When we finally had the mountains behind us, the ride became smoother; the pilot, our hero with the lump in his pants, came on the intercom and said, "Well, we're over the Appalachians okay. Now we just gotta get a look at Newark. In forty-five minutes to an hour or so, on this heading, we should be over it. We'll dive down through this soup and see if we can hit it."

Poor choice of words.

At about forty minutes, there was a yellowish light to the fog ahead of us, indicating a city beneath the fog. Our hero announced, "Hang onto your hat; that must be Newark. I'm going down to take a look."

He dove down through the fog until we came out of it, at about 200 feet above what apparently was the main street. I could read Clark Gable's name on a movie marquee.

A whoop of joy came from the pilot. "Hot damn! See you tonight, honey!"

Poor unsuspecting girl.

After landing, he taxied up to the hangars and we parted ways. I headed for the USO.

"Where can I get a bus for New York City, ma'am?"

"It just left, Sergeant. There will be another one in three hours. Why don't you have a bite to eat, and then we have cots in the back where you can sleep. We'll wake you in time for the next bus."

"That sounds great. Thank you, ma'am."

Her voice sounded like an angel after all that time in the Pacific. She was an angel of the USO, and they were wonderful. They fed me delicious soup and a sandwich, then led me to the cots.

In no time I felt a gentle hand on my shoulder, and a sweet voice waking me up.

"Your bus is here," that lovely voice called.

I thanked them for their kindness and headed for the bus marked New York.

I boarded the bus with a couple of other GIs, and we started off for Grand Central Station. From Grand Central, it was easy to take the train to Springfield, Massachusetts, where I'd take a bus to Camp Devens—back to where it all began.

Camp Devens was an instant reminder of the way the Air Force and Army operated in the States. The usual term was "Chicken Shit," which described all the unnecessary and useless, mindless, rules and regulations that had to be obeyed and tolerated, dehumanizing as they were. It was maddening because the assumption was that the enlisted man could not think and everything concerning him had to be ordered and checked, and he was not to make any decision on his own.

The only Chicken Shit we had had on Saipan happened once. From the Philippines, General McArthur ordered us to put on shirts and long pants despite extreme heat in the planes.

That same day in Washington, General Arnold countermanded that order. What a relief! General McArthur got the message from General Arnold and never came near us again.

Now that I was back home, I could see that army behavior stateside had not changed in two years. Not in the least. The first morning we all were examined, standing completely naked, in a line in front of an officer who was fighting hard to stay awake. There were cursory ear, eye, nose, and throat exams, listening to the heart and chest, a feel of the abdomen and then the mandatory "short arm exam," all performed by a bored doctor, who looked ready to fall asleep at any minute.

We then went through several stations to address different parts of getting discharged. Some were for clothing, others for insurance plans, in addition to the physical exams, which included hearing tests and vision tests.

I got a complete set of Army winter clothes, which I had not had with me in the Pacific (although the quartermasters in San Diego issued us overcoats).

At one table I was given the ribbons for the Pacific Theater battle, with two battle stars, and the standard good conduct medal, and there was another one—I think it was a Victory Medal (for World War II).

At long last I arrived at the final table, the one that inspected our service record and made the determination as to whether we had the sufficient number of points to qualify for discharge.

When I got to that table, a sergeant looked over my records. He looked exhausted and out of sorts. It was around noon time but he looked ready to call it a day.

As I approached him he yawned, gave me a dour look and reached for my papers. Pointing to the empty chair at the side of his desk, he said almost angrily, "Sit down, sergeant."

He leafed through my paper pausing at my MO, which classified me as a Central Fire Control technician.

"What is a central fire control technician?" he asked.

"The armament on a B-29 is all run by computer. That MO is for the technicians who maintain the system."

"Oh." He kept on reading through my record. Suddenly he frowned, turned back to the previous page and then scowled, turned to me and snarled, "You shouldn't be here. You don't have enough points to qualify for discharge!" He acted like he had found a thief as he pointed an accusing finger at me.

Shit.

I had been afraid that this would happen. Immediately I went into my act, which I had given a lot of thought.

"I know that, sergeant, and I tried to tell the captain of my squadron that I thought something was wrong with my points. When I said this, the captain wheeled around and screamed at me, 'you enlisted men are not supposed to think! you are just supposed to obey! Now, about face and get the hell out of my sight, sergeant!' I saluted and hauled ass."

The sergeant listened to this true story. I could see he was getting angrier by the minute. He started to stand up, and got red in the face as he picked up a rubber stamp and said, "So enlisted men are not supposed to think!?" Slam! The stamp came down on the paper. "You just got discharged, soldier." he said and then he turned and shouted: "NEXT!"

After getting my discharge, I caught a bus from Devens to the nearest bus terminal, and eventually stepped out of a Greyhound bus at Jimmy's Smoke Shop on West Main Street in New Britain by Central Park.

How quiet it was! How unhurried! How relaxed everyone was. As I stood there soaking it all in, the South Church chimes started playing hymns, as they did every noon.

I walked around the corner to the bus stop at Central Park and rode the Arch Street bus to the Kensington Avenue drop off.

As I came up that street with my duffel slung over my shoulder, it was a wonderful feeling looking at that great old house, which had been converted from a duplex into a single family home. it was the birthplace of both my father and me. There was a flag in the front window with three blue stars on it. I walked up the slate sidewalk to the porch, went around to the front door, and rang the bell. Mom came to the door wearing an apron, gasped when she saw me, and flew into my arms in tears. There were tears and hugs, touching and laughing, touching, hugging, and kisses all over the place. Oh, how great she felt to me! My mom!

After work, my dad showed up, cheerful and positive as ever, giving me a hearty handshake and a "welcome home, son" greeting.

Then I met Bertha and Thomas, a black couple my dad had hired to help my mother around the house. Thomas gave me a firm handshake and smiled, "Welcome home, Mr. Bob." Bertha just smiled. My mom's parents were living there also, and they were pleased to see me as well. My grandfather shook my hand, and Grandmother looked me up and down for any cracks or splinters; and seeing none, she gave me a kiss, which I had to bend down to get, because she was less than five feet tall. They hadn't changed a bit—just as caring and courteous as ever, and as warm and loving as I remembered them.

My father confided that after paying the $500 scholarship loan, he had used the money I sent home, "… to pay for the help to give your mother a break. However, when you go back to college, you can have power of attorney on my checking account, and you can pay me back for whatever you have used at your convenience." Mother stood there looking lovingly at me.

What could I say? I was going to start my education flat broke, but I wouldn't have had it any other way, and Dad's offer of a power of attorney on his checking account would be very helpful.

PART 4

PREMEDICAL SCHOOL (U.S.)

R emembering my long talks with George on Saipan, I had come home determined to get back into college, and eventually, medical school as soon as I could find a college and register. The decision to "serve God by serving my fellow man" was the driving force in my life, and to this day I have been grateful to the One who so inspired and guided George and me, on that dirt road in Saipan's jungle.

Now it looked liked the only income would be from the "GI Bill," which was $105 a month, plus what I could earn summers, with Dad's checking account as a back up. It looked doable.

As scores of veterans returned from the war, eager to seize the opportunities being offered, colleges struggled to accept all of them who were qualified and who, by virtue of the GI Bill, could now afford to go.

That single bill did more for the American servicemen, giving them the chance for a higher education, than anyone ever imagined it would. Without a doubt, that bill changed the lives of thousands of veterans who were able to go to college or get technical training because of it.

The University of Connecticut, responding to the demand caused by the huge influx of returning veterans, opened a branch in Hartford. The first semester was in Hartford at night, and all the students were returned servicemen. My friend Eaton "Rip" Riley used to travel back and forth from New Britain with me, and after class, invariably, we had a late dinner at Honiss's Oyster House. I almost turned into a clam. Their fried whole belly clams were to die for. A lot of my monthly $105 pay from the GI bill was spent on clams.

While I was going to the Hartford branch of UConn, I lived at home, and was there when my brothers came home. There was another "thank God" celebration each time one of them arrived.

I started dating Jane again, as I had when we were in high school. I had met her on the football field when I was twelve and she was ten, and we were playing opposite each other. I remember thinking, "I'm going to marry her someday."

That wasn't in her plans, however, and throughout high school we would see each other, but she had a crush on a guy I thought was a real loser. He was 4F and into the black market during the war, and because Jane liked him, I didn't.

I remember one dance when she was my date. She had a gardenia in her hair as she came downstairs in an evening gown with a red velvet top and an ankle-length skirt of white netting. When she came out of her house, she pulled up the skirt and jumped the hedge. I thought she looked beautiful in that dress, and her jumping the hedge did not surprise me one bit. She loved a challenge.

In the fall, Rip and I moved to the campus in Storrs. They were in the process of putting up some temporary dorms called South Campus for the returning vets, but until they were complete, I was in a building called the "Quads."

One night I was struggling over a physics assignment. For two hours I had been studying and trying to answer the questions in the back of a chapter from the physics book. I was totally defeated by it and was ready to give up the ghost when someone outside, shouted: "Fire!" I got up and went to the window and saw the beautiful Brick Congregational church, with white columns and a large steeple. The steeple was ablaze like a huge torch. As I watched it burn, I heard a voice so clearly that I know it was real. "Even though my church has burned down, I am still with you."

I was shaken by the clarity of the message, and if I had any doubts, they were removed at what happened next. I sat down and did the physics problems with ease.

When South Campus was completed, Rip and I were roommates, and we struck up a friendship with an ex-marine named Bill Reardon. The three of us egged each other on about all sorts of situations, like how clumsy we were with girls, how ugly we were, and how unlikely it would be for us to get a real pretty date.

One evening Rip started to tell me how and why he was discharged early. While in the service, he had noticed a lump in one testicle, which the Navy surgeons removed and found it to be malignant. In addition to that, there was spread to the neighboring lymph nodes. They told him that in that situation, his outlook was definitely unfavorable (although not totally so) and discharged him early. He was so matter-of-fact about it, and discussed it like it was a done deal, that we never discussed it again.

One night Rip and I were studying, when down the hall comes Reardon singing "One ball Riley" along with a bawdy lyric. Rip looked at me with a questioning gaze.

"I haven't told anyone Rip, honest!"

When Bill entered the room, Rip said to him, "Never heard that song before Bill, where'd you pick that one up?"

"Oh that's an old Marine one; it's been around forever," Bill replied.

A day or two later I told Bill about Rip, and he felt very bad about it, but I assured him that everything was all right and to forget it; just let's not sing that one again.

Rip and I bought a bottle of cider and let it turn, then hung it out the window on a rope in the freezing air, and enjoyed the liquid that didn't freeze very much. Eventually the whole damn building in South Campus had cider hanging out the windows, and soon it wasn't just our building, but all of them were hanging bottles. A lot of the bottles had a tube in them that reached the bottom, so when the cider froze the liquid in the bottom could still be sucked out.

Writing witty things on the plywood stalls in the bathroom became a competition, and aside from the usual "Kilroy was here," and some artistic pieces, there was some genuinely clever stuff written for all to see and contemplate. "The angle of the dangle is directly proportional to the heat of the meat and inversely proportional to the mass of the ass." That one won the blue ribbon.

When I enrolled at the University of Connecticut, I had at the same time sent out letters of inquiry to the top ten medical schools in North America. In response, I received nine mimeographed letters and one typed one.

That was from McGill University in Montreal. They seemed interested in having me, so I wrote to the Dean, Dr. Hatcher, and asked two questions (assuming other things being equal): 1. How many McGill undergraduates were accepted in their medical class of 125 students, and 2. How many Americans were accepted in each class? The answer was: 50% McGill undergrads and 15% American. I did the math and applied to the Faculty of Arts and Sciences for admission as a third-year transfer student, figuring this gave me a 65% chance of being accepted.

PART 5:

MARRIAGE AND PREMEDICAL
SCHOOL IN CANADA

It worked. I was accepted by McGill University as a third-year student in the Faculty of Science to start in the fall of 1947.

Jane and I had gotten pretty serious, and I asked her to wait for me until I finished medical school. She refused, saying, "I won't wait that long. We will get married earlier, or not at all."

Clearly, Jane was not going to wait seven years for me. I didn't want to lose her, so we settled on June 7th as the big day. She planned on working while I was in college to help pay our living expenses.

I arranged to ask her father's permission on a Sunday afternoon. Jane's father, Jim Baldwin, was an executive at American Hardware and an avid outdoorsman. He was a man's man and a no-nonsense pillar of the community.

Jane and her mother were upstairs. Mr. Baldwin and I were in their living room. The conversation went on for over an hour. When we started talking about the battleship "Missouri," I finally took the dive saying, "Mr. Baldwin, I want to marry Jane."

"Well, Bob," he said "we haven't been exactly blind to the increasing love you two have had for each other, and you have my permission to marry my daughter." With that he shook my hand and the ladies were soon in the living room with us. It was a very exciting and happy moment for us.

On June 7th 1947, we were married in the South Church in New Britain. Among my ushers was my dear friend Rip. He had dropped out of school a semester early because his cancer had returned. He looked gaunt and thin. He was in obvious pain, despite his medicines. He stuck it out for the wedding pictures at the club after the ceremony, and then quietly left without saying good bye.

After a great reception we left for our honeymoon at York's Log Village, in the Rangeley Lakes area of Maine. The honeymoon was our wedding present from Jane's parents.

We were greeted at the door by a smiling white-haired gentleman named Dallas Riddle. He was a typical friendly "Down-easter." He had a ready smile and couldn't do enough for us.

"Welcome to York's," he said, "you are in luck, you know, because the ice went out a week ago. Now just drive your car over to Cabin 21, and I'll show you around and help you bring in your luggage."

He showed us through the cabin, and then when leaving said, "Breakfast is seven to nine. Lunch is twelve to two, and supper is six to eight. Of course, you don't have to dress for meals other than to be comfortable. No ties," he smiled.

At supper time we went over to the lodge and met two other couples, also honeymooners. There were loons on the lake, and their singing at night just fit the tone of the place, woodsy and quiet. Every night we went to bed to the calls of the loons. Every night there was a fire going in the cabin, started by Tony the cabin boy. We enjoyed the romance of the evening with a drink, or time alone in front of the fire. We woke each morning to the crackling of a morning fire set quietly by Tony before we got up.

Dallas suggested, after we had been there a few days, that we might enjoy driving up to the garbage dump at night to watch the bears.

"Don't get out of your cars, though!"

What a sight! Every night there were anywhere up to five huge bears rummaging through the garbage. They totally ignored us, and night after night we sat there enthralled by their size.

Since there were horses for hire there and Jane had had experience with riding, we signed up for an hour one day, and the stable master gave us two horses one more spirited than the other.

Because she had more riding experience, Jane took the feisty one, and I rode the other one. After about ten minutes of the ride, Jane's horse kept trying to turn around, and she was having trouble with him. "Let me try him," I said in exasperation.

As soon as I settled into the saddle, that damned horse turned around, and did not stop until he was in his stall with me still on him, trying to control him.

Jane followed, laughing, as we dismounted and left them in their stalls.

I was so glad the stable master did not see us return, because he had been worried that we would be out more than one hour, and he needed the horses. We had been gone only about fifteen minutes.

That placid freezing lake, the loons, the other honeymooners, nights seeing bears in the garbage dump, the fires in our cabin morning and night, which we enjoyed alone together amidst these friendly people, made for a lot of lasting memories of what was a great honeymoon.

Two, days after our return from Maine, Rip died. I hadn't even gotten to see him, and it just tore me apart. I went to his folks and spent time with them, and when they asked if I would be a pall bearer, I said, "Of course." I contacted Bill Reardon, and he served, too.

I did okay at the church where Rip and I had sung in the choir, but at the cemetery, I just broke down and cried through the whole service. I was so ashamed, but I was not able to control the thought that I was going to lower my dearest friend into the ground and bury him with dirt. His beautiful girlfriend (he called her "The Dragon Lady") was there, as well as many of his young friends, and everyone handled it well except me.

After our honeymoon we moved in with Jane's parents for the summer, and her father got me a job working for Coca-Cola, delivering Coke for the summer. It was pretty heavy work, but we needed every cent to get through the winter months at school. I kept that summer job during our first two years at McGill.

As part of my job for Coke, I was supposed to clean one cooler every week. One week I cleaned a cooler on Church Street in New Britain, in a smoke shop/bookie joint. When I told the owner, a man named Rossi, that I was going to clean the cooler, he looked at me, sneered and said, "Go ahead."

I put my money clip with seven dollars in it and my papers on his counter, and then went to work. When finished, I picked up my papers, but the money was gone. "Mr. Rossi, did you pick up my money by mistake?"

He looked me right in the eye and said, "No."

That money belonged to the Coke Company, so that week, seven bucks was taken out of my pay.

Fall came, and Jane and I took leave of her folks' generous hospitality and left for Montreal. It was a fifteen hour drive to Montreal, and we ate the sandwiches Mother Baldwin had made for us before we left Connecticut. When we finally arrived in Montreal, we headed for the neighborhood near McGill, and found a rooming house there which would serve until we got acclimated.

I spent the day getting organized with my classes and inquiring about married students' living quarters. Jane walked around the city and found the going tough. She was homesick, but never said a word to me about it.

The first thing I did after breakfast on the next day was to head for Dr. Hatcher's office. When I arrived at the dean's office, the sign on the door said, "Norman DuPont Ph.D., Dean of the Faculty of Arts and Science." I went in and introduced myself to Dr. Dupont and handed him my transcript and my acceptance letter from Dr. Hatcher. He studied it for a while and then said, "Mr. Rackliffe, I can't accept this admission. The courses you will be taking have, in many cases, other courses you plan to take as prerequisites."

Jesus Christ! He's cutting my legs off!

"I know that sir, but Dr. Hatcher approved this program for me, or I wouldn't be here."

"Well then, I suggest you see Dr. Hatcher, and give him this note from me. You can find him in the chemistry building."

I took his note and, in a panic, went to find Dr. Hatcher in the chemistry building. That sweet gruff old man with the salt and pepper hair listened, and then wrote a note for the new dean that was a plain and simple directive: "Let Rackliffe take any courses he wants to!" signed: Hatcher.

I presented Dr. Hatcher's letter to Dr. DuPont, and after reading it, he couldn't have been nicer. "All right, Mr. Rackliffe, sign up for the courses you need, and good luck."

What a relief! I picked out the courses that I needed for med school. That night we talked to Jane's folks, and when I told them that I had been accepted for premed, I heard surprise in her father's voice. "I thought you were already accepted for medical school."

"No, Dad, that's the next step."

To his credit, he continued to give us his support, even though I knew he had thought that I was already in medical school.

The change from an American school to McGill in Canada came with some rude shocks. Not only was the school year shortened to start October first and end by the end of April, but, as many of the European universities do, there was never any attendance taken, nor were there any quizzes or exams except the final one in the spring! This was scary stuff, with a new wife and no knowledge of how I was doing scholastically. The one saving grace was that exams for each subject, going back ten years were on file in the library. That information led me to understand how things worked, and I hit that library real quick.

Having gotten the academic program in place, we then inquired about married student housing, which every university was supplying for the returning married veterans. McGill had a large married residence, called Peterson Residence, which had been erected for the Royal Canadian Air Force in Lachine, Quebec. It consisted of a group of converted barracks and a mess hall. There was rail service to Montreal ten miles away. Unfortunately for us, it was full, and we were waitlisted.

Eventually, we rented a room while waiting to be accepted at Peterson Residence. The rent came with cooking privileges, and the couple who was renting the room was Mr. and Mrs. Crooks. Their name was very appropriate

He was a beaten old man who said nothing at all, while she was a commander and controller. We were allowed to eat our breakfast when they were through and the same with dinner. There was a frying pan on the stove complete with copious amounts of cold grease that was **not** to be cleaned. The radio in our room could be on, but we were not allowed to increase the volume enough to hear it. I'm sure that our room rent was equal to what they were paying for the apartment. We ate out a lot.

We finally were approved for the married students' quarters in Lachine, Quebec.

We packed everything into our old automobile trunk, which at one time had adorned the luggage rack on an automobile. It was decorated with chrome corner hardware and chrome latches. I put the trunk on my shoulder and walked down three flights of stairs to the vestibule leading to the front door. As I turned to close the door, the edge of the trunk hit the valve stem on the radiator and sheared it off. Water poured onto the tile floor of the vestibule. I went out to ring the doorbell to have Jane come down, but the doorbells were so far from the vestibule that I was locked out. Finally she buzzed the door and I got back in and put my finger over the water leak. I had nothing on hand to plug the water flow, so

I went out and rang again. Jane rang again to let me in. I rang again and finally, angrily Jane came down three flights and asked, "What are you doing?"

When Jane saw the problem, she raced to our room and to get a golf pencil and a knife. I quickly whittled the pencil so that I could jam it into the pouring radiator.

We tossed our things into the car, and then left, walking through the water in the front vestibule like two thieves in the night. Bye-bye Mr. and Mrs. Crooks. So much for you and your greasy frying pan!

My brother Don and his wife Lu drove up with a bunch of old furniture in one of Dad's trucks, so when we arrived at Peterson Residence, we were ready, in a crude way, to set up our two rooms. We had a double bed we bought for four dollars from the Meriden Auction Room, chairs and tables, and a couple of lamps. It sure was nice of Don and Lu to do all that driving for us.

When we first arrived at Peterson Residence, Jane and I found our barracks, and then walked in to the central corridor to our new home. The married students' quarters in the RCAF barracks had been converted into two-room apartments with no running water. The building was in the shape of a capital H, and we found our unit at the end of one of the legs of the H. It was two freshly painted rooms with newly polished floors—beautiful! Walking down the leg towards the cross bar, we met our neighbors John and Isabelle Dixon.

"Hi! We are the Dixons. Welcome to Peterson!"

"Hi to you, too. We are the Rackliffes; Bob and Jane. Happy to be here and to meet you."

"You'll love it here, everyone is so friendly," said Isabelle. They were from Alberta, and John was a surgical resident at Montreal General Hospital and the Royal

Victoria Hospital, which were both in the McGill University group of teaching hospitals.

I could see the look of happiness on Jane's face.

We continued our trip down to check out the bathroom facilities. Jane said that the women had stalls for toilet and shower needs but open area sinks. The men's bath facilities were unchanged from what they had been. Everything was open except the toilets.

All told, that made sixteen apartments per floor, and there were two floors. Everyone there was a veteran, married, and many had children. There was a happy friendliness in a tremendously cosmopolitan atmosphere. We met people from all over the world. On one ski outing, we had two South Africans, one Dutch girl, two Americans, two Australians and one Canadian. We got along famously. The most striking feature of Peterson Residence was the atmosphere of confidence and happy expectations by all the inhabitants. Intermixed with the undergraduate inhabitants, were Ph.Ds, MDs and post graduate students who were studying to attain Ph.D. status.

After Don and Lu left, we put things together in our apartment and then walked over to the mess hall for supper. The hall was filled with benches and tables about six to eight feet long that had been left by the RCAF, and the food was buffet style. Serve yourself.

We helped ourselves to the food, which looked good, and looked for a table to sit down. One young couple waved to us and gestured for us to sit with them.

"Hi! I'm Tom, and this is Mary McFeat. Why don't you join us? You look lost."

"Well, thank you; we are sort of lost. We just arrived. I'm Bob and this is my wife Jane. What faculty are you in?"

"Science, I'm studying geology," said Tom, "and you?"
"I'm premed."

The mess hall was noisy with kids running around and everyone talking at once, but there was an air of cheeriness there.

The cost of staying in Peterson Residence was $100 per month per family, which included one imperial quart of milk per day, pre child. Now considering that GI Bill gave me $105 per month, it was doable with just a little extra money. I am certain that all the numbers were carefully arranged to be affordable for the veteran students by the University.

After a couple of weeks, we knew all three of our neighbors in our section of the "H." The couple across the hall from us was John and Eleanor Dixon. They had been given a bed by a relative, and since it was better than the one they had, they put it up right away. The first night in it, it squeaked so badly that there were three couples out in the hall, cheering on the rhythmic squeaking of the new bed. This brought a red faced, smiling Dr. Dixon to his door in his bathrobe. He asked, "Does anyone have any tongue blades?" These were supplied, a loud hammering was heard and then—silence. This brought on a noisy round of applause.

Most of the students walked down to the train station in the morning to go to the University in the city ten miles away and returned by the same route at night fall. Upon return at night, it was usual to see a line of baby carriages lined up along the lee side of the buildings. There could easily be seven or eight carriages with bonnets up and weather shield over the body of the carriage, even when it was snowing. It was amazing to see them at temperatures well below 20 degrees without a sound out of any of them. They were very healthy and happy babies. I can't remember any seriously ill child. While living at Peterson I recall only one sick adult, Sheila Antrobus, and she had appendicitis, diagnosed by Dr. Dixon.

Sheila was from South Africa and had such a strong English accent she could hardly talk. I drove her to hospital, and all the way she kept apologizing for being "such a bore" while her lantern jawed husband, Toby, said nothing but clamped down very tightly on his pipe.

Jane and I made friends with the Robbs, Ken and Tommy. They had two children a boy John and a daughter Kathy.

One Sunday, John, age four and very dirty, wandered in to the nearby Episcopal Church, where his parents were attending service. He pushed open the door to the center aisle and walked down towards the front of the church. In the midst of the sermon, the priest stopped and looked at the urchin. Ken and Tommie sat there, horrified.

"What is it you want young man?" asked the priest.

The sturdy young lad with one sock down and a mud smeared face said, "I came to see Jesus."

There was silence and then a little laughter as Ken and Tommy quickly got up and escorted their little crusader from church.

Ken was a Canadian while his wife ("Tommy") was Welsh. She had a fiery temper, and Ken told the story that when they were courting, he told her that she had a fanny like a duck, whereupon she wheeled around furious, and socked him in the face. It turned out that "fanny" in Wales meant female genitalia and not the rear end as it does in the States and Canada.

With all those smart people living in one place and with all of them just getting by financially, it was interesting and clever to see how they coped. A group of us went to St. Sauveur one weekend to ski. The owner offered beds in the halls with screens around them as his cheapest beds. We took all of them.

Ingenuity was commonplace. Doug Barron, an engineering student, and his wife had four little boys. They owned a Morris Minor, which was a small English make sedan. With four little boys, I thought Doug was "spot on" when he drilled a hole in the back floor and connected a tube and funnel through the floor to the road beneath. I'll bet it saved a lot of stops.

Another resident of Peterson, a dental student, bought a washing machine and dryer for each building, and anyone who wanted to use them had to sign up and pay him when he came around each week to collect.

I don't think anyone ever cheated him.

A few of the ladies with artistic talent sold paintings, others crocheted table mats and still others sold items they knitted.

Many of the wives, like Jane, worked.

When I started my third-year premed, we were comfortably settled at Peterson Residence. I started on my weird concoction of courses only with the blessings of Dr. Hatcher. This was a heavy load, but I thought I could handle it until I walked into my first class of advanced physics. The professor was young and, in the European style, was wearing a black gown. He had an example on the board on how to calculate the moment of inertia. Every time he added something to the board he would say, "Obviously, then x = y to the tenth power" or some equally unobvious thing, so that after fifteen minutes my stomach was in a knot, and I was totally lost.

I hadn't a clue!

I waited to see him after class, and he couldn't have been nicer. When I told him I didn't understand a word he had said and I thought I was in over my head, he replied, "That's no problem, old chap. We'll just transfer you to first year physics."

Next day I went to my first class in first year physics and was seated alphabetically, which put me next to a big six-feet-plus guy with a huge grin and a warm hand shake as I sat down next to him. I knew I was going to like him, and I think he felt the same towards me. It's funny how sometimes you can sense that.

He introduced himself as Ted Waugh and said he was from Montreal, but had transferred from Yale to be with his father after the death of his mom.

His father was the professor of pathology at the med school, and they lived right on campus. We developed a wonderful friendship, frequently playing squash at noon break. We usually followed that with lunch at his home. The lunch was either made by him or by Rosie the maid, who took care of the house and his father.

After Ted met Jane we became even closer, and there was a constant set of dates, always with another girl in order for Jane to render an opinion. He was fascinated with our living in Peterson Residence, and our being married was something he seemed to feel that he should be doing too, but he was not sure which girl was the right one. Many times we would meet him and the woman of the hour at his house and chat with Dr. Waugh, prior to going to football games in the stadium, which was right behind his house.

Jane's observations were always carefully neutral but interestingly, he eventually married one of them years later, one whom Jane had told me she thought was very nice.

Jane had gotten a job as the secretary to the minister, Angus DeMille Cameron, at The Unitarian Church on Sherbrooke Street. He was young, smart, and full of fun, and his wife was just as much fun and as charming as he was.

In March of our first year in Montreal, Angus invited a minister from Florida to give the sermon one Sunday. Now March in Montreal is not summer—not even close! The guest preacher stood up in the pulpit in a white Palm Beach suit and proceeded to tell the congregation that the greatest example of love ever was Edward VIII giving up his throne for the woman he loved.

You don't say that to Canadians. They considered the duchess a social climber, and a divorced one at that. As for King Edward, he was scorned as one who failed to do his duty. The greetings after the service at the door were, at best, perfunctory.

I wondered how many more Americans were in that congregation and as embarrassed as I was.

One of the medical students who lived at Peterson Residence, Roger Johnson and I were having a chat at dinner one evening when he dropped a blockbuster. He told me that every year six or seven third-year premed students were admitted to the faculty of medicine, and at graduation received both their MDCM and BS degrees. This sounded great: a way of cutting off a whole year of required pemed courses! Next day I applied for early admission in the office of the medical school.

About two months into the third year, we premed students were invited to hear the dean of the faculty of medicine give a lecture entitled, "What to Do When You Don't Get into medical school." His words were ominous.

"There are three thousand applicants for the class of one hundred twenty-five students. Given equal grades the determining factors will be in the following order: 1. Parent a McGill physician, 2. Parent a physician, 3. Parent a McGill graduate, 4. Parent(s) college graduates, 5.Financial ability to pay, 6. Other Considerations."

!!!!!!!

Neither of my parents had gone to college, and in fact, my mother didn't even finish high school. I could not believe that what my parents had done or not done could, or should, affect me.

I decided that it wouldn't. This is how I filled out my application:

> Father: The honorable Fredric O. Rackliffe, a graduate of Princeton University
> Mother: Mabel Foster Rackliffe a graduate of Vassar College
> Financial Resources: Unlimited.

At the oral interview required for admission the members of the board asked me only one question. "What does 'The Honorable' stand for?"

"My father served in the Connecticut State Legislature for eight years," I replied.

That was that. "You may go, Mr. Rackliffe."

Phew! A huge feeling of relief surged through my body.

I received notice the next week that I had been selected to be one of the class of 1952. Jane called her parents and told them the good news, which pleased her parents enormously. It certainly made me feel better, knowing that I hadn't let them down.

I called my parents, too, announcing that there was going to be a physician in the family. They did not seem surprised, but were congratulatory. Mom spoke from her extension. "I am so proud of you, Bobbie!" Dad got on the phone and said, "Well done, son!" That made me feel especially good.

I have always wondered how large a part Dr. Waugh had in that decision, since he was on the board of admissions and knew both Jane and me very well. I suspect his being on the board was a huge help.

PART 6:

MEDICAL SCHOOL

M ed school opened in late September, and within a month of starting classes, I had applied for a scholarship loan from the Kellogg Foundation, despite our "unlimited" resources. These were essentially gifts of $500 to medical students who were in need, and we fit the description perfectly.

On the first day, I wondered how I would react to the touching and dissection of a human body, all cold and stiff, smelling of formaldehyde and lying there, stark naked, along with forty-plus other corpses, some with their eyes open, staring up at the ceiling. How would it feel to cut into the flesh of another human? Would I throw up? Would I get dizzy, or even worse, faint? I guarantee you I had some bad feelings about this, and looking around the anatomy amphitheater awaiting Professor Martin, the professor of anatomy, I could see I was not alone. There was an air of apprehension in the room.

Dr. Martin lectured his way into the amphitheater from the hall, as he always did. He was swinging an entire upper arm, stripped of flesh, with muscles flapping as he spoke. "Now gentlemen, we are going to start our study of the human body at the shoulder. When we have finished, I expect all of you to be able to name the muscles that form the boundaries of the quadrilateral space at two in the morning, blind drunk, and standing on your head."

He was wearing a lab coat over his shirt and tie and had a black patch over his right eye socket. He looked to weigh about 130 pounds, soaking wet, had graying hair, and wore rimless glasses perched in the center of his hawk-like nose. He had a delightful thick Irish brogue, and there was always a trace of a smile on his face and in his voice.

After his lecture, he led us into the anatomy lab where we were divided into groups of four and assigned to a body. These assignments were for the duration of the course, which would last all of the first year, in contrast to the American medical schools where the course was just six months. Dr. Martin was pleasant and strict, but as we stood in groups at our cadavers, he reminded us that these were human beings and were to be treated with respect.

The bodies were laid out alternating male and female, so that students had easy access for study of the anatomy of the reproductive organs of both sexes.

All along one wall of the anatomy lab there were jars of specimens, one of which was so appalling to me that I remember looking at it in disbelief, wondering how and why anyone would have done this. Contained in a three-foot-tall jar of formaldehyde was a one-inch longitudinal slice from head to toe of a baby boy's body.

I found it difficult to look at the little baby boy. What I saw could in no way be construed as respect. I could just visualize some bastard doing that with a saw, and my only feeling was one of fury. I tried never to look at that jar again.

At the time Jane and I were living at Peterson Residence. We were penniless and happy, along with all the other married students who came from all over the world to study at this prestigious university.

I had been extremely fortunate to be able to buy a set of human bones from a senior, and even had the great luck to find a brain (already in cross section slices). Both the box of bones and the covered bucket filled with formaldehyde containing the brain were stored under our bed when Jane and I were not studying them.

All year long the dissection of the bodies continued by each group, and when something unusual was found in a cadaver, Dr. Martin would gather us around the body and commence a discussion.

"Now here you'll notice that the right lung has been removed from this man. One of you tell me what you see."

"Lots of scar tissue and the bronchi are all closed up," came the answer from one of the students.

"And why do you think that happened?" asked Dr. Martin.

"It probably was removed because he had cancer of the lung," replied the student Dr. Martin had addressed.

Dr. Martin nodded and pointed with his pointer to a solid looking lymph node up by one of the collar bones. "You're right doctor, have you noticed this, how large it is and how rubbery?" He poked it and tried to move it, and it was hard and rubbery. "This is a cancer growing still, and I'll bet you two tulips and a daffodil that when you open this patient's skull, you're going to find more cancer in the brain." With that, he took a scalpel and sliced open the lymph node, and there it was—cancer.

Our cadaver also became a classroom opportunity to learn. His left kidney was not in the upper part of the back on his left side, in the usual costo-ertebral angle, but rather, way down on the brim of the pelvis; an ectopic kidney, perfectly formed, and probably was a good functioning kidney, but in the wrong place.

"Well, doctor," said Dr. Martin, "If this man came into your office complaining of pain down there by his pelvis, what would you think of? Kidney stone? I'll wager you one jar of peanut butter and two spoons, it wouldn't even enter your head unless you remember that you have seen a kidney there before."

So it went all year long, finding oddities, and learning the normal and variations of the normal from this humble brilliant man. It was my good luck to have him for my teacher.

By the end of the year our cadavers were reduced to piles of bones and skulls, so after we were done with our dissections and lessons, they were individually put in boxes and taken somewhere in Montreal to a graveyard where they were given burial rites.

Our other studies included histology, which was the study of human tissue under a microscope. For example, the course showed the difference between cardiac muscle cells, striated muscle cells and smooth muscle cells, and physiology, which was the study of how things worked. An example would be why the pupil of the eye widens, and how it does it when one is frightened.

Additionally, we studied bacteriology, with labs included, so we could recognize the bacteria that cause lockjaw, or the one that causes cholera, along with the many other bacterial enemies of human beings.

In pharmacology, we started to learn how medicines worked and which ones worked for specific conditions.

Toughest of all was biochemistry, which attempted to explain the chemical changes when a muscle contracted and relaxed, and the waste products such a chemical reaction would create, in this case, lactic acid. All in all, it was very demanding, and very fascinating.

At home in Peterson Residence, Jane helped me to learn the skeletal anatomy every night studying those bones. A previous owner had painted nail polish on the bones to show where the muscles attached. Jane spent hours pointing to different parts of each bone and asking questions such as, "what muscle attaches here? What nerve opposes the action of that muscle? Where does the muscle insert? What function does it perform?"

We did the same sort of intense study on the brain, too. Jane and I studied all through the first year every night, with her spending hours helping me learn anatomy. I think Jane learned more anatomy than I did.

Jane became pregnant in the first part of the first year, and her due date was late May. She continued to work at the church through most of her pregnancy.

Well into her pregnancy, in the middle of winter, she developed a craving for a cucumber, and she purchased the only cucumber in Montreal for $2.00. This was an extravagant expense which we could ill afford, but she was so happy with it, how could I object? I was delighted that her obstetrician was Dr. Sparling, because all the medical staff and students said he was the best. Jane loved him!

One wintry night during her pregnancy, Jane left to go to medical wives' club at Mr. Dodds's home. She was so late getting home, that I was relieved when I heard her coming in. "Hi," I said, "I was beginning to worry about you."

Jane burst into tears.

"I had an accident," she sobbed.

"Was anyone hurt? How did you get home? What happened?" My questions came in rapid fire.

"No one was hurt, and Mr. Dodds brought us home. I was trying to get up the hill to the Dodds's house, but it was too slippery, so I was backing up to get a better start and I backed into a streetcar. They had to tow the car away."

"Well, thank God, you're okay. Don't worry; every thing will come out all right. Let's go to bed."

Next morning, Jane was sitting at the table as I got dressed and she said, "There's something I didn't tell you."

"What?"

"I wasn't driving. Some man from Vancouver was. He and his two friends were in Montreal for a convention, and they saw us trying to get up the hill, and they were trying to help us by pushing. Finally one of them, Mr. Stirling, suggested that we get out and the three of them get in to make the car heavier. So two of them got in the back seat and Mr. Stirling drove."

Jane continued. "He asked the guys in the back seat if anything was coming, saying: 'I'm going to back up and get a running start.' The rear windows were totally fogged up so one replied, 'I can't see anything.' Mr. Stirling took that as a 'No,' and backed down into a main street and right into the street car."

Jane continued to cry.

"That's okay, honey, we'll get it fixed."

"But that's not all," she sobbed.

Jesus! What else could there be? "Tell me," I said.

"Mr. Stirling told me to tell the police that I was driving because it was an American license plate."

"Well, that won't do. Do you have a local number and his home address?"

"Yes, I do. He's staying at The Mount Royal, room 234."

I called him in the hopes that at seven o'clock he would still be in his room. He was.

"Mr. Stirling, this is Bob Rackliffe, and I am calling you about last night's accident. First of all, I want to thank you for trying to help my wife. It was very nice of you to try and help the ladies out."

"I'm so sorry about the accident, Mr. Rackliffe. When George in the back seat said he couldn't see anything, I thought he meant that there were no cars in my way and I was OK to back up. I didn't realize that he really couldn't see because the windows were steamed up."

"I understand that completely, Mr. Stirling, and I want to emphasize that I am most grateful for your attempt to help. However, I think it would be an error to leave the police thinking that my wife was the driver, so I intend to correct that statement, and I just want you to know."

An air of hostility became immediately apparent. "So you're going to put the blame on me, is that it?"

"No, not at all. I'm simply going to tell the truth, and I don't see anything to worry about, especially when I talk to some gallant French policeman about my wife being pregnant. I'll just say she had to say that because it was her car. I just wanted to thank you personally and give you a heads up about the correction that will be given to the police."

"Well, thank you for calling, Mr. Rackliffe, and again, I am very sorry to have caused this mess." The phone clicked and he was gone.

The desk sergeant answered the phone on the second ring. "Westmount Police Headquarters, Sergeant Gagnon speaking."

"Sergeant, this is Mr. Rackliffe speaking about the accident at 9:00 p.m. last night on St. Catherine Street, when a car was hit by a streetcar. Do you have the case available?"

"Just a minute, Mr. Rackliffe. Ah yes, your wife was the driver."

"Actually, Sergeant, she wasn't. She is pregnant and thought that since we owned the car, she had to take the responsibility for the accident; you know how pregnant women can be, sergeant—"

"Oh oui, monsieur, I understand. Do you have the name of the real driver?"

"Yes, it is Mr. Gordon Stirling. He is staying at the Mount Royal, but I don't want any charges brought against him. He was just trying to help."

"*Tres bien*, Mr. Rackliffe, we will make the corrections and close the case."

"Thank you very much, sergeant."

Next, I called my dad and told him what had happened.

"Get it fixed up, and when you know the price and are ready to pay, I'll put the money in the account so you will be covered." Dad was cheerful as ever and so supportive. It was such a comfort to me to have him backing me this way, but he was always upbeat, and much more so since I was in medical school.

"Thanks, Dad."

The bill was a hefty US$875. I had them make out two estimates.

I sent one of the estimates to Mr. Stirling in British Columbia with this note.

> Dear Mr. Stirling,
>
> I want to start off by thanking you again for your attempt to help my wife when she was in trouble. As you know, I am a medical student, and money is very scarce in this vocation. If it is at all possible to help us with this bill, we sure would appreciate it. If that is beyond your means, do not concern yourself with it. I am grateful you stopped to help my wife.
>
> Signed,
> Bob Rackliffe

I showed this letter to a law student friend of mine at McGill, and he said, "You've cut yourself right out of ever getting anything! You've ruined your chances."

About a week later I received a letter from Mr. Stirling.

> Dear Mr. Rackliffe,
>
> When I got home from the convention in Montreal, I told my wife what had happened and we decided to cash in some bonds and mail you the money that we can afford. I'm sorry it can't be for the whole thing.

It was signed, Douglas Stirling.

In the envelope there was a check for $400.

Mother Baldwin came up to be with Jane in time for her due date, 20th of May.

That brave woman slept on the sofa in the living room, used the toilet facilities in company with all the other women, helped Jane with the wash using the pay washing machine in the ladies part of the "H," and never complained once. She was a brick.

Final exams for the first year were scheduled for the last week in May. Jane went into labor on the thirtieth of May late in the day, so the histology final which was in the morning was safely done. That left the worst subject of all, biochemistry, the last exam on the first of June.

When Jane went in to labor on the afternoon of the thirtieth, we two ignorant first-timers called Dr. Sparling, practically with the first contraction, and he ordered her to go to the hospital. So I took her straightaway to the Catherine Booth hospital in Westmount. This was a maternity hospital run by the Salvation Army and was originally for unwed mothers. It was still for unwed mothers, but they also took married women as well. It was a wonderfully happy place, as most obstetric floors are, and with all those babies being born, why not?

She was examined and put to bed. They were confident she would not have the baby any time soon, so they medicated her with something. I don't know what, but it was as if someone had thrown her "wake up" switch to the "On" position. Jane became irrational and kept getting out of bed to "go to the church," or to "fold the laundry," or "to go to dinner," or for no reason at all. She was perpetual motion and had to have someone in attendance at all times.

It was the student nurses, Mother Baldwin, or me, who got the duty, and it went on until 7:11 a.m. on June first when Master James Palmer Rackliffe entered our world, and at 9:00 a.m. an exhausted mother was in a deep sleep, while an exhausted father seated himself in class for the biochem exam.

And what an exam it was! We were presented with two complex compounds and were required to demonstrate the chemical reaction that would take place, producing a third compound which we were supposed to name and describe its properties.

I started out logically enough and demonstrated a fair degree of knowledge of the subject, but somewhere I got lost and ended up with a compound totally foreign to me. So I wrote, "I'm not sure what this compound is but I'm sure it would explode! Enjoy the enclosed cigar; my son was born at 7:11 this morning."

I passed the course with a B.

In the fall of that year, the professor told the new freshman, "My final exam was so tough last spring that one of the men had a baby."

After Jimmy's birth, Mother Baldwin stayed around to help for about a week and then headed home, much to the joy of Dad Baldwin, who didn't like living the bachelor life.

Just two weeks after Jimmy was born, we packed up and started on our fifteen-hour trip home to New Britain, Connecticut, with Jimmy in the back seat of our little coupe, comfortably tucked in on a mattress that just fit in the space behind the front seat.

Arriving at the international border, we were stopped by the Canadian authorities, who asked me to open the trunk for their inspection. After finishing their look in the trunk, he spotted Jimmy in the back seat.

"Where'd you get the baby?" he asked.

"My wife had him at Catherine Booth Hospital in Montreal," I replied.

"Do you have proof of that? Do you have any papers?"

"Copies of his birth certificate were not finished at City Hall in Westmount when we left. What's this all about, officer?"

"There have been a number of Canadian babies sold to Americans in the last six months, and we are stopping that traffic, that's what." He glowered at me.

This was getting scary. "Look, officer, I am a medical student at McGill University and this is my wife. That is our son, born two weeks ago at Catherine Booth Hospital. Why don't you call them and confirm what I am saying? Besides, my wife is breast feeding him, so it's not likely that we would have bought him, is it?"

He walked around the car and noted that we had both Connecticut and Quebec license plates on it, then he came up to me with a little smile, looked at Jane, and smiled at her, and said, "Well, Doc, if your wife's nursing, and your car is registered in both Quebec and Connecticut, I'm inclined to believe you, so congratulations to both you and the Mrs., and have a safe trip home."

"Thank you, officer."

We had no trouble at American customs, just a stop long enough to show our U.S. residence address and proof of citizenship, and we were off.

By this time Jimmy was really howling, so we drove a while to the border and went off to a quiet deserted road so that Jane could nurse him. We arrived at Jane's parents' home around ten o'clock at night to a very excited grandmother and an interested grandfather. Dad put his index finger in his namesake's hand and smiled, as Jimmy's hand tightened on grandpa's finger.

We stayed with them for the summer, and Jimmy had Jane in fits with colic, until one night she had a Manhattan about twenty minutes before she nursed him.

He slept the night away and that sort of got everything straightened out.

I worked for Coca-Cola again that summer. By September, I was anxious to get back to school. Mother Baldwin fixed us up a lovely group of sandwiches and fruit and cookies for the fifteen-hour trip. Goodbyes were sad and tearful as we started our trek back to Montreal.

Mother Baldwin's lunch was eaten before we left Connecticut, and all through medical school, her lunches never made it out of the state.

Second year was in sharp contrast to the first year of medical school. First year was all laboratories and lectures, and no patient contact. From sophomore year to the end of the fourth year, we would be studying and learning with real patients. The subjects to be covered in the remaining three years were medicine, surgery, obstetrics and gynecology, urology, pediatrics, pathology and psychiatry. We would not perform any procedures such as spinal taps, or starting IVs at all. This was in marked contrast to American medical schools, where first year students were doing all these chores. At McGill, it was felt that those techniques were supposed to be learned in the intern year. The years in medical school were to be spent at all times with a professor in attendance.

The first morning as we started learning the subject of medicine (which would be a three-year course), I was in a group of five students, all with bright and shiny stethoscopes around our necks, our professor, the soft and gentle white-haired Dr. Milstein, looked approvingly at our white coats and said, "Gentlemen, today we are going to study the effects of rheumatic fever on the heart. This disease, which is an aftermath of exposure to streptococcal infections, causes the valves in the heart to be scarred, contracted and covered with vegetations along their edges, so that they leak, and thereby weaken, eventually causing death. These changes in the valve function produce a characteristic sound in the heart that can be heard with a stethoscope, thus confirming the disease. For some reason, females with fair complexion, particularly redheads, are more prone to this disease, and the patient we are to examine is a red-headed female."

By this time, we were standing in a group alongside a bed that was obscured by drapes. Opening the drapes and ushering us in, Dr. Milstein then closed the drapes and said, "Doctors, this is Miss Martin, who has kindly consented to let you listen to her heart, so that you can hear the murmurs of mitral stenosis and mitral regurgitation. You will please watch me listen to her heart, and follow my demonstration carefully."

Miss Martin's bed was cranked up about fifty degrees, and she was covered with a "Johnny coat" put on backwards so the front could be opened. She was a very pretty strawberry blond of about twenty, and when Dr. Milstein bared her chest, her face reddened noticeably, she got the undivided attention of the young docs.

Dr. Milstein then examined her heart for a long while, pointing out those areas where the murmurs could be heard best, he gestured to Mike who was next to me on the right side of the bed to have a listen.

Mike bent over and placed his stethoscope on the inside part of the left breast as the Dr. had done and carefully and slowly moved it across her breast, which made the pink nipple stand up as he reached the side towards her armpit. He took a long time listening as he went. The rest of us watched in rapt attention, as his hands moved over her chest.

Quietly, after what seemed like five minutes, Dr. Milstein said, "Doctor, I think you would hear the murmurs better if you put the earpieces of your stethoscope in your ears."

The poor girl turned even redder as Mike hurriedly plugged in his stethoscope, and once again toured over the breast listening to her heart, and then retired sheepishly to the foot of the bed. Mike was redder than Miss Martin.

There was no smiling or any inappropriate behavior as the rest of us took our turns listening to the murmurs, but after class when we were alone, Charles Rally was all over Mike. "Cheap feel, eh Mike? Boy! You sure looked stupid!"

Psychiatry was studied at the Allen Institute of Psychiatry. It was a palatial estate with beautiful grounds on the banks of Mount Royal, adjacent to the Royal Victoria Hospital and the university. At our first lecture, the chairman of the department, Dr. D. Ewen Cameron walked up to the lectern and said, "Welcome to the study of psychiatry, gentlemen. One of the first things I want you to understand is that you are never to display any surprise, approval, or disapproval of anything a patient says. For example, if a patient says to you, 'I am so mad at him I could kill him with an axe!' your response should be, 'that's interesting, why an axe?'"

He then continued the lecture on the theme of it being necessary to be non-judgmental.

A few days later, it was a lovely spring day, and I decided to bring my lunch to the Allen and eat it out on the beautiful grounds. After the morning lecture and discussion, I was sitting with my back against a tree, facing down towards the main path to the house. There was a squirrel the other side of the tree from where I was sitting. I was trying to entice him into taking part of my sandwich, talking to him and gesturing. When Dr. Cameron came up the path, the squirrel was not visible to him; I was embarrassed at what the doctor might think, so I said, "There's a squirrel behind this tree."

'Of course there is." He replied with absolutely no expression on his face; no interest, curiosity or doubt. Nothing.

Non-judgmental all right, I thought to myself, and went back to the squirrel, which promptly bit my finger, grabbed the piece of sandwich and took off.

"Ungrateful little bastard!" I said, and sucked my bleeding finger.

About a week later the class was assigned to the psychiatric ward at Montreal General Hospital, and the doctor in charge walked down the hall with us, assigning patients to us as we went. Nodding to me, he said, "Doctor, I want you to go into room 223 here and interview the patient. His name is Charlie, and I'll join you in a half hour or so."

So I went in and greeted Charlie. "Hi, Charlie, I'm Dr. Rackliffe. How are things going?"

"Just fine Doc, and thanks for asking."

"Are you married, Charlie?"

"Yes, I have a lovely wife and two great kids. Matter of fact, my daughter is in her first year at McGill," he replied.

"How old is your son, and what's he up to?" I asked.

"He's sixteen and in high school, and a heck of a hockey player, if I do say so."

"What do you do for a living?" I asked

"I work for Eaton's in housewares," was his reply.

The remainder of this very pleasant conversation gave me no clue that he was anything but normal and a nice guy at that. There were no grimaces, noises, or unexpected behavior the entire time I was with him.

In comes the professor. "What do you think, Doc?"

"Seems fine to me," I replied.

"Is that so?" said the professor, then to Charlie, "So Charlie, what time are the bombers coming over today? Three o'clock?"

"Nope," said Charlie with a smile, "they'll be here earlier to surprise you."

Our obstetrical rotation consisted of lectures in the morning, then supervised clinic in the afternoon. These were prenatal clinics and post-natal checkups. Each of us had to spend one week in the hospital at night to deliver any ward patients (patients being attended by the students or house staff) that might come in and deliver. If there was an emergency of some sort, such as bleeding, a resident or intern would be there with us.

In the afternoon clinics, we each had five or six ladies assigned to us. When they came in for checkups, we were called, and in the best-case scenario, we would deliver them while we were on our in-hospital rotation.

One of my patients was a very lovely French lady named Belanger. I had examined her twice at clinic in two weeks time because she was near term, and I had noticed that she had a mole on her right labia about one half inch in diameter.

The week I was on call to deliver any of my classmates' babies, I was called to the delivery room and told to get there in a hurry. After putting on a hat, scrubbing for ten minutes, then a gown and finally gloves, I entered the labor room. I advanced toward the foot of the table towards the patient already in the stirrups and draped, so that the only flesh showing was her vulva.

There was a half inch mole on the right labia.

"Ah ha! Bonjour Madame Belanger! C'est moi—Docteur Rackliffe!"

"Oh bon! Bonjour, Docteur!"

In my fractured French, the conversation went on as the baby started to come:

"Desirez vous un garcon ou une jeune fille?"

In perfectly understood English came the reply.

"I don't give a damn, docteur, just as long as it gets out damned soon!" This was followed by a huge strain and grunt, and a baby boy was in my hands.

Perfect he was, and his doctor was prouder than the boy's father.

(I wonder happened to that baby and where he is today.)

Back at Peterson residence, things were going well, so well in fact that Jane was pregnant again and due in the middle of August 1951. We were delighted, but I'd bet a fig or two that her mother wasn't looking forward to staying in that two-room apartment with the public showers and toilets again.

Jane was active in the medical student wives' club. They would meet once a month at the twelve-room mansion of Jackson Dodds, whose married son was a medical student one year behind me. Mr. Dodds' home was on the top of Westmount Mountain, just west of Montreal.

He was a very famous man, having been general manager of The Bank of Montreal, which had branches across Canada. His picture was on the five dollar bill in Canada. His son Donald's wife and Jane became very good friends.

One night in my sophomore year, Jane came home from a meeting of the wives' club and said, "Mr. Dodds wants us to come to tea Sunday. He said to bring the baby along, too."

"Why? What's up?"

"He didn't say, except he wanted to discuss something with us. I told him we would be delighted."

When we arrived on the top of Westmount and rang the doorbell of this imposing house, we were led into the front hall by the butler. He asked us to wait there a moment, and almost immediately a tall white-haired man appeared from another room and greeted us.

"Come in! Come in!" he called cheerfully with a huge smile on his face. "And this, his hand on Jimmy's head, is the heir apparent. Well, Ruth will take care of him, perhaps take him for a walk, if that is all right with you, while Hutchins serves us tea."

A woman following Mr. Dodds smiled and said, "I'm Ruth, and I would just love to take your son for a walk in our stroller. Is that all right with you?"

Jane smiled and said, "Thank you, Ruth, he would love that. I'm sure he won't give you any trouble." So Ruth popped him in a stroller, gave him a Lorna Doone cookie, and off they went.

Mr. Dodds led us into the drawing room and seated us in two overstuffed chairs, one on either side of his, arranged around a coffee table. Hutchins came in shortly thereafter with tea, cream, sugar, and some tea biscuits.

After a short while, Mr. Dodds explained why he had asked us for tea.

"I have a proposition for you. I am leaving for Europe on the tenth of June to attend a Boy Scout meeting in Austria. On the first of August, I will return home for one night and the next day. Then I'll be heading out to the west coast for another month with the Boy Scouts of Canada. Of course, it will be in the papers, and I am concerned that an empty house will be a temptation. I wonder if you would consent to spend the summer here? It's good for the help to have someone as a guest of mine here, too. You've met Hutchins and his wife Ruth, but there is also a gardener and laundress. They will purchase all the food and, oh by the way, there will be a gross of eggs delivered the first of every month. I will be returning the last weekend in August. What do you think?"

He stopped and looked at us, and smiled.

Jane and I looked at each other. I think we both thought immediately of her mother and what a difference this would make for her comfort when she arrived for the new baby.

Jane answered Mr. Dodds. "That is a very generous offer Mr. Dodds, but I have to tell you that my mother is coming up prior to my delivery date in mid-August, so we can't impose on you to that extent."

"Well, Jane, she certainly is welcome here when you will need her the most. There's plenty of room. I don't see that as a problem," Mr. Dodds replied.

"In that case, Mr. Dodds, we will accept your invitation, and thank you for considering us. We will plan on moving in for the summer on the fifteenth of June."

This was more than just a break, it was a godsend. Peterson Residence had closed, and we were in student housing at MacDonald College, the agricultural campus of McGill. It was twenty five miles from Montreal. The married students' quarters was a series of tarpaper-shingled condominiums with one bathroom between every two two-room apartments. We cooked our meals on a two-burner hot plate and shared our bathroom with a family of five.

Because it was the agricultural college of McGill, there were plenty of vegetables and fresh fruits for the married students. It was ordered that only windfalls could be taken, but many were the nights that the guard would have the ladies hold his light while he shook the tree for "windfalls."

On June fifteenth we started our life in a mansion in Westmount with the neighbor on one side named Bronfman (who owned Seagram's Liquors) and on the other someone named Timmons, who had discovered a gold mine. They had a chapel on their premises with a pipe organ in it, which was played every Sunday.

We arrived about 2:15 in the afternoon, and were greeted by Hutchins and Ruth, who helped me in with all the baby equipment and showed us to our room. The room was very nice, having enough room for Jimmy's crib, and also had its own bathroom. In an hour or so we were all unpacked and moved in, so we took Jimmy downstairs with us to look around. There was a screened-in porch off the huge dining room, and Hutchins suggested we go there and have tea, which we did.

"Dinner is usually served at seven, but Ruth thought that maybe with the baby you would rather have it earlier, Mrs. Rackliffe. What time is suitable for you?" asked Hutchins.

Jane replied, "First of all, while we are here we would rather be called by our first names, Hutchins, and secondly, Ruth is right. Six p.m. would be much better for us because of the baby. So, it is Bob and Jane please, and may we call you by your first name, too, or would you rather we didn't?"

"That is fine with me Mrs.—er, Jane. But when Mr. Dodds is here in the mid-summer, it'll have to be Mrs. Rackliffe; I hope you understand. You can call me Hutchins, though; I am so used to it, and it is fine with me." He smiled and looked a trifle more informal.

"Fine!" said Jane, "I'm glad we got that straightened out."

We went out for a walk around the neighborhood after putting Jimmy down for a nap; we eventually ended up on the screened porch reading the paper.

At 6:00 p.m. the dinner chimes sounded, so we made our way into the dining room and put Jimmy in his high chair (a Baby Tenda, which was a little table with the baby seat right in the middle of the top so that he could not drop anything on the floor, nor could he tip it over). The dining room table was fifteen feet long, and Jane and I were sitting at opposite ends so neither of us could reach Jimmy, and he needed to be reached regularly, so Jane moved her place alongside his, and that's the way the table was set from then on.

After we had finished dessert, Hutchins asked, "Would you care to have your coffee on the porch?"

"That sounds fine, Hutchins. Thank you." So we moved onto the porch and that too became a habit during our stay.

Next morning I went off to the anatomy lab where I was going to be doing some research every weekday morning, and odd jobs in the afternoons if anyone called the university for a student to help. That first afternoon, I went home at lunchtime because there were no odd jobs for me.

Lunch was set up for us in the dining room, which was all Jane needed to see. She marched into the kitchen and asked Ruth, "Would you mind if Bob and I ate lunch out here with you and Hutchins? We're just not comfortable in there and would really rather be with you and have someone to talk to while we eat."

"Of course not, Jane," said Ruth.

From then on we had lunch in the kitchen with the Hutchins.

"Bob," said Hutchins "would you mind if I took a couple of outside jobs during Mr. Dodds's absence. Of course, you mustn't tell him, or I'll not take the jobs, but Ruth and I could use the extra money."

"That's fine with me Hutchins, go for it."

So for the rest of the summer, both Hutchins and I were laborers until the gong rang for dinner.

Mother Baldwin arrived by plane the last part of July and was comfortably accommodated awaiting the big event.

She was there for the weekend when Mr. Dodds arrived and for the dinner he shared with all of us on the one night he was there. We were all spiffed up for dinner, and Mr. Dodds took his rightful place at the head of the table.

"How was your trip to Europe, Mr. Dodds?" Jane asked.

"Very well thank you, Jane. It was an international meeting of the leaders of the Boy Scout movement, and as the representative of Canada, I was quite busy. It was grand seeing my old friends from all over the world, and I have a lot of information for the meeting in British Columbia that starts tomorrow. Has every thing here been going well here?"

"It has been just wonderful, thank you so much."

"And you, Mrs. Baldwin, are you comfortable here? Is there anything more that we can do for you?" he asked Mother Baldwin.

"Gracious no! You've been so kind to the children!" she replied.

We had tea on the porch and spent an hour or so in small talk, and after a while Mr. Dodds rose and said,

"Please excuse me, but it has been a long day for me, and I think I will retire. I will be out of here early tomorrow morning before you are up and about. Good luck with the new baby, Jane."

We said good night, and thanked him again for his hospitality as he left for bed.

Throughout his brief stay, we were all shining stars of decorum, much to Hutchins's relief.

Jane went into labor on the seventeenth and delivered our second son on the eighteenth of August. The delivery was much easier than the first, and we named him Dan Eaton Rackliffe. ("Eaton" had been my dear friend and college roommate Rip's first name.)

As soon as Ted Waugh heard the name Dan, he rushed up to Catherine Booth Hospital and hung a large picture of "Handsome Dan," the Yale bulldog, over Jane's bed. There were many and loud protests about this from the student nurses, but Jane laughed at Ted for his constant teasing.

Dad Baldwin arrived in late August to see the baby and pick up Mother Baldwin. They said their good byes to Hutchins, Ruth, and Jimmy, Jane and me, and headed out towards the Thousand Islands and the Wisconsin Dells on a long-planned vacation.

On the thirtieth of August we had tearful farewells with Hutchins and Ruth, and headed back to our two-room home in St. Anne's. Boy! What a shock I got when I started to pack our little coupe with a small back seat! I couldn't believe that two such little humans needed all the stuff they did. Somehow I got it all in, and we squeezed into the space that was left, leaving our mansion on the hill for our place in St Anne's, which seemed like "Tobacco Road."

The intensity of senior year was compounded by the demands put upon us by the kids. Jane was nursing Dan, so of course two-year-old Jimmy needed to be taken care of by me a lot of the time. The routine became one of kids first. When they were in bed, study time was next and consisted usually of study from 8:00 p.m. to midnight, then tea with Jane and then to bed. The only normal nights (i.e., no studying) were Friday and Saturday. In all the years of study we never compromised. Friday and Saturday were fun days.

I had been attending lectures on diseases or systems like the cardiovascular system since second-year medicine. Every once in a while the lecturer would go out of his way to make the point that his lecture was important. Whenever that happened, I would make a big star on the notes. I did that religiously for the three years of classes, so when I started studying for final exams, I studied all the starred lecture material first and made dammed sure I knew those subjects. In contrast to the undergraduate schools, there were no copies of previous years' exams for medical school.

Clinical hours were spent, mostly afternoons, in the four hospitals. The Royal Victoria crowned the top of Mount Royal, and loomed over McGill University like a jealous old maid. It was rivaled in size only by The Montreal General Hospital, which was down in the city proper at a much lower level geographically, and in the opinion of the "Royal Vic" staff, educationally. Nestling on one side of the Royal Vic was Montreal Children's Hospital, which like a child looked up at the grand dame. On the other side of Tthe Royal Victoria was the prestigious Montreal Neurological Institute—a seven-story building specializing in neurological problems and neurosurgery.

It was here one day that seven of us sat in an over-hanging observation booth, looking directly down on the brain of a man whose skull cap had been removed so that the whole top of his brain was exposed. The famous neurosurgical pioneer, Dr. Wilder Penfield, sat at his head with a little probe and asked the man where he felt the probe. (Amazingly, this procedure was painless to the man and he was fully conscious.)

"You are on my left knee, Doc."

Dr. Penfield explained to us that the man had a form of epilepsy (Jacksonian), wherein prior to each seizure he would have a feeling in his left big toe. Dr. Penfield was trying to locate the left toe area on the man's brain

"Now where do you feel?"

"Inside left ankle bone," came the reply from the man.

A little move of Dr. Penfield's hand.

"And now?"

"You're on the big toe, Doc. That's it."

Zap! Dr Penfield hit the area with an electrocautery, and then spoke. "We're all done, Paul, and I think your problems will be over now. Dr. Ingram will finish up here." Then turning to face us and taking off his gloves, he said, "What we have done here, gentlemen is to ablate [destroy] the area from which his seizures have started. I wish it was always this easy."

We stayed a little while longer to see the man's skull put back in place against the bone from which it had been cut. Then the scalp flap which had been hanging off the back of his head was put back in place and sutured together, covering the skull. (This too was painless as the entire area had been injected with local anesthetic.)

The week of final exams came, and one after another, the questions in almost every specialty were the ones that I had starred over the last three years. The result was predictable; I had done very well. So well in fact that at the oral exams in the afternoon, I was quizzed for about an hour, and then dismissed with instructions not to leave, but to wait to be recalled. *What the hell is wrong?* I asked myself. The student following me in the oral exam, Charles Rally, came out of the exam looking as frazzled as I felt and sat down by my side.

"What the hell is this all about?" I asked him.

"I have no idea at all," said Charles.

"Mr. Rackliffe, please come in," ordered the dean of medicine, standing in the doorway.

"I want to put a question to you, Mr. Rackliffe. Suppose you were called to see a fifty - year-old thin woman who is in heart failure, and has had diuretics, morphine, and digitalis, and is still in failure. What would you do next?"

"I'd order thyroid studies."

"Why?"

"Because it is one of the chief causes of lack of response to treatment of congestive heart failure."

"Thank you, Mr. Rackliffe, you may go."

A while later Charles came out and we left together. Charles was exuberant. It turned out that the extra oral exam was to determine who would get the medal for best in medicine, and the doctors had congratulated Charles. I did, too, and I was pretty proud of the fact that I came in second. I only wish that I had known the real purpose of the second oral. I thought this was to see if I had passed the course. It never occurred to me that I was in a race for the medal.

Overall, I finished second in medicine, and tenth in general standing in the class.

This was the first class since 1927 where every one of the men admitted to the class four years earlier graduated. It was called a "White Glove" class, and tradition was that we would present of pair of white gloves to the dean of medicine at the graduation ceremony.

I will never forget the looks of happiness and the joy in the hallway as the marks for the year were posted and everyone graduated. It was a special moment for all of us!

Driving back to St. Anne de Belleview, I was thinking of how much of this was due to the efforts of Jane, and how those efforts would go unrecognized for so many veterans' wives who had put up with years of privation, scrimping, and going without the nicer things in life, just to help their men, because they believed in them.

I wrote my feelings about this to Dr. James, the Principal of McGill University, and sent the letter to him, hoping that he would pick up on it and give recognition to the wives of the graduates at the commencement. At the commencement ceremony he read my entire letter, without mentioning its source, as his tribute to the "silent partners" of the graduating class.

It was great to see my mother and father, who came up for the graduation and sat with Jane. The boys were being baby sat at McDonald by a neighbor. When my name was called, and I went across the stage, Dr. James shook my right hand and handed me my genuine sheepskin diploma from his left, winked, and said, "Congratulations, Doctor."

Jane presented me with a sweep-second-hand wrist watch which she had gotten from a jeweler in New

Britain, promising to pay him $5 per month 'til it was paid for.

I had nothing to give Jane except a promise that some day I would take her to Lake Louise in the Canadian Rockies, the prettiest place on earth.

We did go to that breathtakingly beautiful place, many years later.

PART 7:

INTERNSHIP AND RESIDENCY

A few days after graduation, my brother Don and his wife drove up to Montreal in a three-ton stake truck, which we loaded with all our furniture (including the four tea crates), and we headed home. When we got to the border, the American inspector asked, "What's all the stuff on the truck?"

"That's our furniture."

"Hell, Doc. Now that you're a doctor you should just have junked this stuff in Canada,"

"On an intern's pay of $95 per month, that stuff is going to see a lot more service before we can throw it out," I replied.

When we arrived in New Britain where I was going to intern, Don and I carried all the stuff up to the second-floor apartment that would be our home for two years. One of the maintenance men built us a kitchen table out of a piece of used plywood, which was all we really needed.

While I didn't start my internship at New Britain (Connecticut) hospital until the first of July, we were allowed to move into the second floor apartment of a three-family house a week early. It was right behind the hospital; lovely, roomy, and airy. The rear entrance to the hospital was about one hundred fifty feet across a parking lot in the rear of the house.

Chris Steinmayer was the chief resident in medicine, and since that was going to be my first rotation, he was selected to show me around.

"Well Bob, let's get you some uniforms, so you'll look like all the rest of the monkeys here." He said that without a smile and in a resigned air that suggested a dry sense of humor. We went to the laundry room where Chris introduced me to Bertha, who was in charge.

"Glad to meet you, Doc," she said. "what are your sizes?"

"Probably large, I think, Bertha. Could we try them for fit?"

"Of course. Go right into the linen room there and close the door," she said as she handed me trousers and a jacket.

When the fit proved to be right, Bertha loaded me up with six uniforms, so I turned to Chris and said, "Lead on, captain, and thanks, Bertha."

Chris smiled. "Now let's go to the treasurer's office, and you can find out how great the pay is."

We met one of the younger administrators named Al, who was about my age. Al was also was living in back of the hospital with his wife and two daughters.

"Hi, Bob! Glad to meet you!" he boomed. "Now let's see, you are coming in as an intern (first year), so you will be earning $95 per month minus $41.50 for the apartment. Of course, your laundry is free and so is the food. That sound all right?"

I allowed as how it was, since that was the going rate at some hospitals. At the university teaching hospitals, pay was even worse: $25/month.

When we left his office, Chris said, "Don't worry about the food, Bob. When you come over for dinner tonight with your family, have them stand behind you in line, then load up your tray with all the food for the family, and don't be bashful! Everyone does it. You'll see."

So that night, Jane and I made our entrance to the dining room of the hospital, and as ordered, stood in line with Jane right behind me telling me what to take, while the two boys got the silverware and glasses and then waited for Jane and me to finish and pick out a table.

Loaded with what looked like a week's worth of groceries I moved my tray up to the cashier and looked at her.

"Welcome to the hospital, Dr. Rackliffe, we are glad to have you and your lovely family with us." She smiled as she eyed the amount of food on my plate.

"Thank you," I replied, and as I started towards a table in the dining room, another resident called out and said, "Doc! Pull in here!" as he gestured toward a table next to theirs, complete with a high chair.

When we pulled in there, he stood up, proffered his hand and said, "Hi! I'm Charley Goyette, and this is my wife Natalie, and these are our two kids, Christian and Amy."

I introduced Jane, and we sat down next to them and had a pleasant dinner with the Goyettes. Following

Charlie's lead, I went back for a tray of desserts (with a lot of assistance from Jimmie and Dan). The boys loved the unlimited ice cream.

After dinner we walked over to our apartment, which filled Jane with joy. It had been freshly painted and was huge! There was a kitchen big enough to have a table in it, around which we could all sit and eat if we wanted to stay home for dinner or for breakfast. It was equipped with a refrigerator, and there was room for our washing machine, too. Off the back porch, there was a clothesline on a reel. Directly off the kitchen was a dining room, living room, and two bedrooms and a bath. This was a palace compared to the two rooms, hot plate, and shared bath in Canada!

Jane was so happy with it she said, "I can't wait to make some curtains and get them up."

Monday morning I went over to the hospital, had breakfast with Chris, and waited nervously for what would come next.

We started the morning with rounds, which was a tour of the medical floor, presenting the ward cases to the attending physicians. Ward cases were those patients without a private attending physician, and they were our responsibility.

Frequently, with the consent of the patient, private cases were presented, too, especially if they had a unique or rare problem.

The senior attending physician of the month was Dr. Ed Resnick, who happened to be a graduate of McGill, too.

"Glad to meet you, Bob, and please feel free to call me any time if you have a problem."

"Thank you, Dr. Resnick; I appreciate that very much because I feel very green at this."

"Don't worry about anything, Bob. You are well-trained, and it will all fall into place for you."

That was reassuring. All morning (and every morning) rounds were held and long discussions about EKG appearances, lab results, and x-ray interpretations were the rule at all of these rounds. I was occasionally called to the ER in the middle of rounds, but aside from that, my job was to present the case and the problems and listen to the comments and orders for future tests.

Afternoons were mostly taken up with doing procedures on patients and admitting new patients. This consisted of a lengthy history and a thorough physical exam. I enjoyed being on the lookout for some thing or condition for which the patient had not come into the hospital but, nevertheless, was medically significant.

Every morning before medical rounds, I would do nursery rounds, and the ward babies were my responsibility (including circumcisions). I would talk to the moms every day and discharge them when ready to go home.

Someone had scheduled a circumcision for the first morning, so I asked Chris to show me how it was done.

The baby was strapped to a board, and the only part visible besides his face was his penis, and that looked pitifully small for starters. Nevertheless, Chris sterilized the field with a cold antiseptic solution, draped the baby with a sterile drape that had a hole in the center for the penis, and then said to me, "Okay, doctor, pick up the mosquito forceps and slide the point down between the foreskin and glans. Good. Now slide the point down to the level of the crown of the penis. Okay. Now open the forceps."

Opening the forceps separated the foreskin from the glans in one easy move.

"Now slide the pointed end of your scissors between the foreskin and the glans down to the level of the crown;

that's right, now cut it." I did, and a small amount of blood came out, but the baby didn't even cry.

"Now Bob, take a hold of each side of the cut foreskin with a gauze pad and peel it back from the glans, so that it is entirely loosened from the glans."

I followed his directions to the letter. At this point he handed me a Gomco clamp, which consisted of a little bell on one end of a T-shaped bar. The bell part was put over the penis and under the foreskin, after which the T-shaped bar was brought up through a hole in the bottom of the clamp to a receiver for the T part. As this was tightened, it drew the penis upward, crushing the foreskin, which always made the babies cry briefly. All that was left to do then was to cut the foreskin off that had been pulled up with the bell, and the job was done. A Vaseline gauze dressing was applied, and that was that.

"Good job, Bob!" said Chris wryly. "I don't know why you are sweating."

At five o'clock all the house staff who were not on-call left, and those of us who were on-call stayed at the hospital. Jane came over with the boys, and I ate with them, being paged twice during dinner. When dinner was done, I kissed her goodbye, and headed for the emergency room. I was a wreck! What if someone came in who was in diabetic coma? What if a kid came in with croup? What if someone came in convulsing? My head was whirling with all the horrible things that were coming in for the doctor to cure, *and I was that doctor!* Jesus Christ!

Just as we finished dinner, I was paged for the emergency room.

"Hi, doctor, this is the ER secretary, and Nurse Washington wants you to come by at your earliest convenience."

The head nurse greeted me. "Hi, Dr. Rackliffe. I'm Marie Washington, and I am the head nurse of this zoo. It's Harry Hopsmith. He's in congestive failure and he comes in more and more frequently. He is an employee here."

"Is he on digitalis?"

"Oh yes, has been for over a year. Usually when he comes in like this he gets a shot of morphine and an intravenous diuretic, along with some oxygen, and he's good to go by morning."

I went over to Harry's bed, smiled at him, and said, "Hi, Harry, I'm Dr. Rackliffe, and I am here to see if we can get you straightened out. Let's have a listen to your chest."

I helped him up to a sitting position and listened to his lungs, and there was no doubt that he was in congestive failure. He also had edema around his ankles, which indented when I pressed on them with my thumb.

"I'm having trouble breathing, Doc," he panted.

"I know, Harry; we're going to fix you right up."

Nurse Washington arrived with a syringe of morphine, and pushed an IV stand for me to start my first IV. Fortunately, Harry had dandy big veins, and I had that IV going in nothing flat, as if I knew what I was doing.

With Harry taken care of, I spotted one of the surgical residents, Bert House, and asked him if he was busy.

"No, Bob, what can I do for you?"

"Teach me how to tie a surgical knot with one hand."

"Piece of cake," he said, and in a matter of minutes, he taught me the little moves that made knot-tying so easy. "Take some suture material up to your room tonight, Bob, and practice on the bed post."

So until midnight at least, I was either tying knots on the bedpost or looking up in my pediatric and internal medicine textbooks as to what to do if some other emergency came in that night.

Chris went out of his way to teach me all the manual techniques required for the job, such as getting blood samples, spinal taps, lung taps, and liver biopsy by needle aspiration, cut downs, etc. I have to say I hurt a lot of people while I learned, but I guess every doctor out there has done the same.

Dorothy Slater was a constant complainer and in hospital an abnormally frequent number of times. On this admission, Chris said, "You know, Bob, I think Mrs. Slater is faking her sudden onset of complete paralysis in her legs and weakness in her arms. I think a lumbar puncture is in order, and this is the perfect time for you to do an LP."

Okay. This would be a first. Four of us lifted obese Dorothy onto the table and hauled her on to her side; I sat my gowned and sterile self on a stool behind her. After sterilizing her back with a cold brown solution, I then injected the area with a liberal amount of lidocaine. Holding the four-inch-long lumbar puncture needle in my right hand, I probed her back with my left hand trying to feel the spine of a vertebra beneath which I planned to insert the needle into her spinal canal.

I could not feel a spine, but inserted the needle where I thought there would be one. Nothing. All the way in and no spinal fluid. Missed!

Beads of perspiration were on my forehead, and a thoughtful nurse wiped me off.

I made another attempt to feel the needle pop through the sheath of the spinal cord. Still nothing. Another miss.

She was so fat! Looking or feeling for a vertebral spine was hopeless. It was like Pin the Tail on the Donkey, and her obesity was the blindfold.

Two more tries and a miracle happened. She got up off the table, erupting in a fountain of foul language as she walked out of the room. "Fuck you, Doc! What the fuck do you think I am, a fucking pin cushion?!"

Chris watched her go with a dour smile on his face and said, "Well Bob, you cured her paralysis."

Late one afternoon, I was paged almost non stop until I answered. "Doctor, you are wanted on pediatrics right away," said the operator.

"Okay, thanks."

There was no doubt in my mind that this was an emergency from the way she had paged me, and from the way the operator spoke.

Lois Winterville, the head nurse, met me at the door, and took me to a side room where, sitting up and leaning forward (an ominous sign of air hunger) was a beautiful blonde haired little boy named Christopher, of about twenty months. His anxious parents stepped aside for me to examine him. When he tried to breathe in, his chest would cave in toward his spine, his nose would flare, and the sound of the inhalation was very labored and noisy. When he exhaled there was a pronounced wheeze and a huge effort on his part to breathe out, as well as in. It was like trying to breathe through seventy-five feet of garden hose. Lois said his temp was one hundred two degrees. After I listened to his lungs with a stethoscope, it was immediately obvious that very little air was moving, despite his labored breathing. The lungs were full of wheezes and moist rattles as he labored.

I turned to the parents. "This little guy is in deep trouble, and I want to call for an Ear, Nose, and Throat consultation immediately. He needs a tracheotomy and the sooner the better. This will involve cutting into his trachea, and inserting a cannula into his trachea or windpipe. That will make it easier for him to breathe, and allow us to suction the mucous out of his lungs more thoroughly. He has a disease known as Respiratory Syncytial Virus, or RSV. It is a disease of infants and young children, and can be serious."

"Whatever you say, Doctor," the Hendersons answered in unison.

In twenty minutes or less, a doctor showed up and announced, "I'm Dr. Norman Johnson, an associate of Dr. Daley." Dr. Daley was the chief of ear, nose, and throat at the hospital. Dr. Johnson went right to work after the parents went to the waiting room. We scrubbed as a nurse opened up a tracheotomy set from Central Sterile Supply. I helped him as he performed the "trach."

While he was operating, he said, "I'm new here. This is my first week with Dr. Daley."

"Me, too, Dr. Johnson, this is my first week, too."

"Call me Norm please, Bob, I don't feel comfortable yet as an attending surgeon."

"Okay Norm, but you sure know your stuff the way you are going now."

Once the tube was in place, we suctioned Christopher out and put him in a high humidity oxygen tent. His respiratory rate decreased considerably and he went to sleep almost immediately. He was exhausted.

Although he was better, neither Norm nor I felt comfortable about leaving him, so we stayed on. As the night wore on, Christopher's condition worsened, despite suctioning and IV Cortisone. He continued to struggle as his teary-eyed parents tried to comfort him. The longer the struggle went on, the feebler were the poor little guy's efforts to breathe. At about seven in the morning, God took his little hand in His and they left together.

To this day, more than fifty years later, I can still see that sweet little boy struggling to survive, recall the moment he left, and feel the sobs of his mother on my shoulder as I watched his father, tears running down his face, staring at the lifeless body of his son.

As the year progressed, I found myself drawn more and more to pediatric medicine. It was "medicine with hope," whereas on the internal medicine floors, there was frequently an air of acceptance of death as an inevitable part of life. There were many occasions when letting the patient "cross over" was an act of kindness to relieve pointless suffering.

I felt that this was the proper way for an internist to think. I saw no merit in prolonging the inevitable when the case was hopeless. With children, it was different. They had their whole lives in front of them. I liked the idea that given good medical care, a child who was desperately ill could, by virtue of his young age, be saved to live a long life. This was a young body, not some tired and worn-out old person and there was the difference and the challenge.

I wanted to hurt when I lost a child, and I always did. This was not the case with adults for me. I could appreciate when the outlook was hopeless, and so be relieved for the suffering patient when he finally died, but frequently, medical care prolonged the agony to the inevitable end.

For example, take the case of the seventy-two-year-old Polish immigrant factory worker. He was admitted to the medical floor on the ward service with widespread metastatic cancer involving his liver, brain, and lungs. He was going to die. All of his life in America he had worked at the Stanley Works, bought and paid for a three-family home, and saved a few dollars. Ward service meant that he was a "teaching case" and the doctor on ward service would not send a bill, but would oversee the care of the patient managed by the house staff. The doctor on ward service that month was the chief of medicine, Dr. Snowman.

This looked like an easy case to me. Our job was to keep him free of pain until he died. Period. It would not be a long time and would require only simple care; inexpensive care. However, Dr. Snowman had different ideas. "Doctor, I notice his electrolytes need to be corrected. Please see to that, and in addition, get a liver profile."

"But, doctor, he is riddled with cancer and will not live more than a few days; why waste his money on tests that are not going to affect the outcome?"

"Because I ordered it, Doctor. I want this man to die in electrolyte balance. Do you have any other questions?" His eyes leveled at me were cold and challenging, poised to strike.

"No, sir," I said, and looked directly into those evil eyes in disgust.

Two weeks later, after innumerable IVs and an astronomical number of lab tests, and about $75,000 poorer, the man died in agony, but in electrolyte balance.

Mentally, I compared this death to Christopher's.

Another example that soured me on practicing Internal Medicine was that of a lady admitted to the private floor with a diagnosis of anemia. Her anemia was Pernicious Anemia, which explained her hemoglobin of 2.5 grams (normal being 12–14 grams for a female).

She was given two units of blood immediately, and despite the fact that she was a Christian Scientist, she did not object to the transfusion (which she said was against the beliefs of her religion). Every day I went in and started a transfusion without objection from her, until her hemoglobin was back up to 8 grams and she was beginning to feel pretty good. Then she began to speak out. "You know, transfusions are not an acceptable form of treatment for a Christian Scientist, and I wonder if I should continue to have them."

Finally, when her hemoglobin was up to 11 grams, she signed herself out of the hospital against advice of her physician.

Her doctor, an older and wiser physician, just smiled and said, "She'll be back before the year is out, Bob. Her religion is directly proportional to her hemoglobin. The lower her hemoglobin the less Christian Scientist she is, but the higher her hemoglobin gets the more devout she becomes."

Dr. Foley was a bear of a man. He was a true general practitioner. Everybody loved him, and he loved everyone back. He never lost his humility. He would say, "When I get over my head, I just call the experts." There weren't many times when that was the case, because he was a pretty sharp and experienced doc, but he did just that. Whenever he had a case he thought was beyond him, he would call in a specialist. One day he called me from his office. "Bobbie, I'm sending in a guy I think you know. He is in diabetic coma, and I'd like you to handle it. If you get in over your head, call me, and we'll get a third doc to look in."

Hot Damn! My own case and a hard one! I did know the guy; we were the same age and had been in school together since elementary school. He had always been sort of a swaggering wise ass. He hadn't been in the war because of his diabetes. He was a car salesman at the time of admission.

He was, as Dr. Foley said, in a deep diabetic coma. I used all my newly learned talents to bring him round so that by the third day, he was sitting up in bed and eating again.

"Bob, Dr. Foley told me that you saved my life and I want to thank you. Whenever you need a new car, look me up, and I'll take care of you."

He took care of me all right. About four months after he left the hospital, I went over to his automobile dealership to look for a real good used car. First thing he looked at was my old car and said, "This is perfect! This model is in great demand, and should give you a great price on your turn-in."

Then he showed me a nice used car and said, "I think we can get you in this car for your turn-in and $300."

This sounded too good to be true, and it was. The manager refused the deal, and the counter offer was $800 and my car. And I, like a fool, took the bait, when I should have walked out.

This is called "low balling" by car salesman, and involves giving an unrealistic appraisal to the car being turned in, and then having the manager put the kibosh on the deal when the customer is hooked on the car to be purchased. How stupid of me! My old car had never given us trouble since we had driven it, new, home from the dealers.

This kind of adult treachery and duplicity was making me wonder about taking care of adults for the rest of my life. Really! I had saved the bastard's life, and he returned the favor by screwing me!

One Saturday night I was in the hospital cafeteria when I was paged. It was the hospital operator calling to say that a man had suffered a shotgun blast and was on his way in to the operating room. The shot had been to the abdomen. They were getting the surgical team ready for him. I was to go to the OR at once and start scrubbing.

I gulped down two sandwiches and a coke, and took off for the OR to await the ambulance bringing in this challenging case.

Upon arrival at the hospital, the guy was in pretty tough shape, unconscious, IV drip going full out. A hoard of nurses, orderlies, anesthesiologists, surgical techs, lab techs, and doctors were all present and working to get him quickly to the OR, where we were prepared and waiting.

The patient was a nasty person who had a long rap sheet of assaults, robbery, and drugs. He had been shot by a relative, who stood at the bottom of a stairwell, shotgun in hand as the patient stood menacingly at the top of the stairs. He got the entire load of shot right in the abdomen.

When we opened him up, there were pellet sized bleeding points everywhere: liver, intestines, ureters, kidneys, bladder, and especially, his aorta. every organ was bleeding. We were suturing the holes while he was getting unit after unit of blood. About four hours later after he had had six or seven units of blood and our blood bank was becoming exhausted, the anesthesiologist said, "If this bastard dies now, I'll kill him!"

He died while receiving the last unit of blood in the bank. His body was sent to the morgue with a bunch of instruments sticking out of his hastily closed abdomen. The pathologist would return them to central supply when he did the autopsy. We had started at 6:30 p.m. and we finished at 2:00 a.m. Everyone was exhausted, and I'm sure most of us felt a little defeated at the loss, however worthless the man.

When I left the OR suite, there were seven calls waiting for me. One of these calls was from Miss Gilmore, a student nurse. "Doctor, would you please come up to S-306 and catheterize Mr. Mullins? He has not voided since surgery this morning." When I got there, Miss Gilmore helped me put on a sterile gown and sterile gloves. Then she drew back the bedcovers and prepared to remove the urinal from between the patient's legs.

It was full.

"Oh my!" she gasped, and looked at me with a guilty little grin. She looked so cute, standing there with a urinal full of urine and as red-faced as I have ever seen anyone. I took off the gloves, looked at her and smiled. "Goodnight, Miss. In the future, please check the urinal first. Now I'm going to bed and I'm counting on you to let me stay there." I'm certain she expected to hear more than that.

By the winter of my first year at the New Britain General, I had pretty much decided that Pediatrics was what I wanted to do, so I went to the chief of staff and told him that, but that I had made a commitment to the chief of medicine to do a year there as junior resident in medicine in 1953, so what should I do?

His response was immediate and to the point. "Bob, we want you to be happy. If that is the way you want to go, go with our blessing."

So I applied to Henry Ford Hospital in Detroit for a residency in pediatrics, which boasted one of the finest residencies in the country.

About a week later I was summoned to the administrator's office.

"Bob, I received a letter from the Ford hospital in Detroit informing me that you are applying there for a pediatric residency. Is that right?"

"Yes, sir. I cleared it with the chief of staff, and he encouraged me to go into the field that I really want, and I really prefer to go into pediatrics."

"But you are already committed here for a year in internal medicine, and I don't think you will get released from that."

"Look, Mr. Knight. I'm already behind because of my service in the war, and I have a wife and two kids. I don't want to waste a year here. Besides, the chief of staff gave me the okay to apply."

"Well, I'm sorry, Bob, but I will not release you unless Dr. Snowman goes along with it, and that's final."

Dr. Snowman was even nastier. "You agreed to stay here as a second year resident in medicine within two weeks of your arrival here. I will not release you from your contract."

"But, Dr. Snowman, as I told Mr. Knight, I am already behind three years because of the war. I have a wife and two kids. I don't want to waste a year here, doing something that will be of no help to me."

"Doctor," he threatened, leveling those cold snake-like eyes at me, "if you do not fulfill your agreement to spend the year here, I will have you blackballed in every hospital in the state."

To my dismay, the chief of staff did not speak up on my behalf.

There was no choice for me then, so I determined to spend as little time as possible on the medical floors, and when on-call at night, to seize every opportunity to get that bastard Dr. Snowman out of bed or, at least, awake. Whatever it took, I would do it, to keep him annoyed and short of sleep. I swore I would spit on his grave. I studied all of his cases in hospital and wrote many progress notes on his patients' charts, calling attention to deficiencies I noted, questioning orders that were not medically indicated; anything to annoy him or embarrass him. I have to say though, that there were not many mistakes; he was a pretty good internist, even if he was a son of a bitch.

Meanwhile, the chief of pediatrics, Dr. Ros Johnson, called me within forty-eight hours of Dr. Snowman's threat, expressing his shock at the action and said, "Bob, I will meet you every morning at seven and do rounds with you all year."

He did that. Every morning I had at least an hour of his teaching and he even opened the door to all his private patients, as well as the other pediatricians of his group, in addition to the ward cases, so that I was seeing twenty to thirty sick patients a day with him right at my side, sharing his experience with me on a one-to-one basis. He had a tremendous pediatric background, and his partner, Dr. Crothers, had studied pediatrics at Yale, and was also a good teacher as well as a friend.

During that year I managed six cases of meningitis, several severe dehydration cases from diarrhea, and many cases of worm infestations. Several children with fevers of unknown origin were given to me to handle, and all in all, it was a wonderful year for learning with a good variety of patients.

I have always been grateful to Dr. Johnson for doing what he could to correct a rotten situation. As for the chief of medicine, I never spoke to him again (except on those occasions when I could wake him up). The silence was deafening when walking past him in the corridors of the hospital with no one around except the two of us. I detested him, and he knew it.

Meanwhile, Jane had undergone surgery for varicose veins, and her legs looked just great, when she announced we were going to have another baby, due in August of 1953; two years after Dannie, almost to the day. She was her usual cheerful, caring wife and mother all through the pregnancy, and was at term one morning when I left for work at the hospital on a beautiful August morning.

Suddenly, over the paging system came the call: "Doctor. Quick! Delivery room! Doctor. Quick! Delivery room!"

My heart stopped. *It couldn't be Jane. She was having little pains when I had left this morning but was not even in the hospital,* I thought, as I ran for the delivery room.

The delivery room was bedlam. One of the mothers in labor was being "quicked" because she had a condition called "Disseminated Intravascular Coagulation," a condition that occurred rarely in pregnancies, and was usually fatal. The cause is unknown, but the result is that the patient starts having small blood clots all over the body, so in short order the elements necessary to form clots are exhausted, which in turn causes the patient to bleed from every imaginable source. Parts of the fetus have been blamed for the onset of the disease.

That was the situation when I arrived in the delivery room, and that was the time I received a call from admitting that my wife was being sent up to maternity in active labor.

All hell was breaking loose in the delivery room where the woman was dying when Jane was wheeled into a labor room. I sat with her and tried to act normally, but I was scared to death! After a while, the noise and number of people in the delivery suite became less, and Jane's hour was fast approaching. The nurses checked her and decided to move her into a delivery suite right next to the one with the door closed—the one with the dead mother in it.

For this delivery, I stood behind Jane and watched as the baby was delivered. The baby's face was so beautiful that I thought maybe it was a girl—the prettiest of all my offspring—but as the delivery continued, evidence soon came into view that changed her sex real quick. A beautiful, healthy, long little boy. And Jane was fine, too! What a relief! We named him Peter Baldwin Rackliffe, the middle name being Jane's maiden name.

After three days in hospital, Jane came home, and there we were with three little boys: Jimmy, Dan, and Peter. Jane and I couldn't have been happier with our sons. I always thought that Jane was a perfect mother for boys, and they were lucky to have been born to her.

When I had started pediatrics, I had promised myself that I would go into practice with someone so that I would be guaranteed time off with my family. I had watched two pediatricians who were in solo practice, and even though they both had children, they were never with them. That was not for me! I was going to be a father with my sons, and Jane and I were going to make our lives revolve around them and enjoy them.

Dr. Greenblatt, a senior pediatrician in New Britain, heard me make that statement when I was doing my residency there. He called me the next day.

"Bob, this is Harold Greenblatt. Your statement interested me yesterday. I have been considering getting into a partnership with someone, and if you are interested, I would like to sit down and discuss it with you."

Now I had been working with this man for one and a half years when this conversation took place, and I had nothing but admiration for him. This was great!

"I'd love that, Dr. Greenblatt. Thank you for asking!"

"Fine. I'm delighted. We can go over a few details in the time remaining this year. Do you need any money to get through?"

"I think when I make the move to the residency in Akron, I might, doctor."

"Well, just let me know, and I will advance it to you."

About halfway through my second year at New Britain, I had applied to Akron Children's Hospital and was accepted for a residency the first of July 1954. This was a great opportunity for me, as this hospital took care of all infectious disease including polio for eleven counties in Ohio. There were one hundred eighty-five beds in this pediatric hospital and a dynamite chief of staff, Dr. James G. Kramer—famous throughout the pediatric world for his diagnostic ability and contributions to pediatrics.

We were to report there for duty on the first of July, 1954. Housing was to be supplied free and the pay was an astounding $400/month plus meals, living quarters, and laundry!

As the year wound down in June, the Goyettes left for Maine, the Browns were staying another year in obstetrics, Chris was going into practice, and the other intern, Betty Hannon, was off to Pennsylvania for a residency in pediatrics. When it came time to say goodbye to Chris, I went over to his apartment to see him, and he was there alone.

"Where's Pam?" I asked.

"Aw, I guess she's pretty well on the way home by now, Bob," he said. Then he looked down at the ground and pushed some dirt around with his shoe tip and added "We're getting a divorce, you know. I guess she couldn't stand me or, what the hell! Who knows?"

"Shit, Chris! I had no idea you were having problems. I'm so sorry."

"That's okay, Bob. I guess I'm not the greatest bargain in the men's department."

"What are you going to do?"

"I'm going to open a practice in Bristol. Probably make a flop of that, too."

"Aw, cut the crap, Chris. You'll do great. I have never seen your equal in the two years I have been here. Don't be so down on yourself. Anyway, I came over to thank you for all you've taught me, and tell you how great it was to work with you and for you." I put out my hand, which he took limply, looked me in the eye, and then quickly looked away.

"Good luck, Bob," he said as he walked away without looking at me.

The next morning my brother Don came over with the big truck from my father's business, and the two of us loaded all the stuff we had trucked down from Montreal onto it and he was going to get to Akron the day after we did.

For the newcomer, entry into Akron is noteworthy for two things: 1. the smell of burning rubber and 2. the smell of oatmeal. I knew it was the home of Firestone, Goodyear, Goodrich, Seiberling, and more tire companies, but I had no idea that Quaker Oats also came from here. The melding of these two odors into one was unforgettable, and I'm sure it caused a lot of sinusitis and allergic rhinitis as well.

We stumbled around in downtown Akron, and finally pulled up in front of Akron Children's Hospital. I entered through the main door and approached a telephone operator I could see through a sliding glass window. When I came up to the window, it zipped open, and a chubby, smiling lady turned to me and said, "Hi. Can I help you?"

"Yes, thank you, I am Dr. Rackliffe and I am one of the new resident staff. Who do I see to get to where we are going to live?"

"Oh, welcome, Dr. Rackliffe! I'm Myrt, and I will get Dallas Winter on the line for you." She rang a number and then announced, "Mr. Winter, Dr. Rackliffe is here. Thank you." She turned to me and smiled. "He'll be right out."

Shortly, a trim, gray-haired, good looking man came hurrying down a corridor, stuck out his hand, and said, "Hi, Dr. Rackliffe! Good to see you. I'm Dallas Winter, and I will show you over to the resident apartments." We went out the front door where he met Jane and the boys and said, "Maybe you had better follow me over, as it doesn't look like we're all going to fit in there. Wait here and follow me when I come by in a green Ford."

In a matter of minutes, I saw his Ford coming at us, when he turned into the parking lot in front of us, gesturing for me to follow him. We went through that parking lot and came out another entrance, where about a half block down on the left, a lovely four-story apartment building came into view. He pulled into the driveway, which it shared with a wreck of a house of the 1890s era, and stopped his car.

"That's the resident and interns' quarters," he said, pointing to the beautiful apartment building, "however, it is full, so you and your family will be on the ground floor of this beauty."

He was pointing to the wreck. What a disappointment! The house looked like something from a murder story in a rainstorm. It was red brick and three stories high, with a very steep slate roof with demon spikes. There was lots of gingerbread hanging from the wrap around porch that had been repaired at the entryway only. It was dirty, and the trim had at one time been painted gray.

The house looked perfect for a reenactment of Lizzie Borden's axe slayings, with spikes on the roof, and snow gates up there, too. Some windows had shutters, some had one, and some had none, and many were not hanging square.

"You'll be living only in the left side of the first floor, as we are planning to pull this down in the future, so only that part has been made livable. I would not want you to go through any other parts of the house, as the floors are not safe."

Front to back there was a living room, two bedrooms, separated by a bathroom and a cavernous kitchen with a pantry off one side and what had been a huge (7'x9') closet on the other side next to a rear entrance.

My brother Don and his wife arrived as planned with our collection of crappy furniture, and our fifty-dollar washing machine in one of my father's trucks. We used the same four tea crates (plywood) that we had had in Canada with circular openings at one end. They were piled up on top of each other for our bureau. Our double bed was still the four-dollar beauty from the Meriden Auction Room. Our washing machine was a riot. Whenever it started to spin, it would start "walking," and the boys would get up and run to hold onto it 'til it stopped, perhaps two to three feet from where it had started. It never failed to make Jane and me laugh to watch the kids scramble to hold on for dear life when it started to spin. We put Peter in the little room off the kitchen and put Jim and Dan in the other bedroom.

Night came, and with it a wind and the whispery breezes throughout the closed part of the old place: noises, groans, banging, creaking, and ghostlike movements of window curtains (in the absence of a breeze). When the furnace came on in the cellar, the old house groaned and crackled. Winter made it worse, but by then we had all the ghosts named.

The noises bothered Jane and me but not the kids; not in the slightest. Kids are amazing! By noon the next day after we arrived, they were playing and friendly with all the other kids. The parents were a different story however. They were cool and very superior, and did nothing to make us feel welcome.

Our attempts to get to know and fraternize with the house staff hit a big bump in the road when two weeks after our arrival, Dan came down with the chicken pox, and suddenly all the kids and their moms were gone from the outside gathering places, and angry stares came our way from the parents. In the weeks to come, many of the residents' kids came down with chicken pox, which didn't endear us to the parents. You would have thought he had leprosy the way some of the wives and their husbands reacted! As a matter of fact, one of the residents accosted me at the hospital to tell me my son had chicken pox. His wife had called him at the hospital and reported it to him. Whatever progress we had made towards acceptance by the senior residents and their wives was lost.

It was obvious to me that generally speaking, senior residents consider themselves the most brilliant and talented physicians they have ever known. In fact, I think it is the point where most physicians are at their most knowledgeable. The only thing missing is experience and a touch of humility.

My first rotation was in the infectious disease ward. The day I entered for the first time, there were six cases of meningitis for me to care for. (I had seen six cases in two years at the New Britain General.) I could see I was going to learn fast. My first week there, I was shown a three-month-old infant by his pediatrician. "'Bob," he said, "this baby is three months old, and his birth weight was seven pounds, six ounces. As you can see, he is only about nine pounds now, and is emaciated. Clearly, he is failing to thrive, and I don't know why. He's been worked up for everything I can think of and even his diarrhea, which is chronic, does not have any pathogens in it. If you get any hot ideas, feel free to do whatever you think is necessary for him."

"Yes, sir, Dr. Swan, I'll give him a thorough look first thing."

Next day I was standing there next to his crib, looking at him, and I percussed his head almost absent-mindedly. The technique is to put the heel of your hand on the upper part of the forehead so that your fingers overlie the skull. Then raise the middle finger off the skull in its entirety, and thump it down against the skull. When you do this procedure, it feels and sounds as though you are tapping a ripe melon on a normal infant's skull. The left side of this baby's head sounded and felt just like that, but the right side felt and sounded like I was tapping on concrete. This was distinctly abnormal!

I turned to the nurse and asked, "Did you hear that, Mrs. Blossom?"

She answered excitedly, "Yes, sir, I sure did. It's different on one side."

"Well, now, we will have to do a subdural tap on the right side. Do we have subdural tap kits made up?"

"The subdural needles are included in the spinal tap trays," she said. "I'll get one right away."

She was back in a flash with a spinal tap tray, and sure enough, there were two half-inch needles (20 gauge) included in the set. After prepping the side of his head with an antiseptic solution, I carefully inserted the little needle in the suture line between his frontal bone and the parietal bone. Thick pus came out! We had our diagnosis. He had an infected subdural hematoma. Subdural hematomas are inside the skull, under the Dura, which is the membrane covering the brain. The hemorrhages are usually caused by a fracture of the skull either by use of forceps or during the birth process as the skull passes through the pelvic rim of the mother.

Infection of these hemorrhages is uncommon, and the cause of the infection was not usually known. They could be completely without symptoms, but could also continue to enlarge and put pressure on the brain with consequences requiring surgery.

We cultivated the pus and notified Dr. Swan, who called a neurosurgeon. The neurosurgeon opened the area by putting in burr holes in two places (about three-quarter-inch holes) to evacuate the pus and instill antibiotics. We added antibiotics to his IV, and over the next two weeks he recovered, gained weight, and finally went home, cured.

Why had I done that percussion? What made me do that? As I reflected on this case, I couldn't explain why I had done it, so clearly, as I would find throughout my medical career, there were times when I did things I couldn't explain that turned out to be exactly what was needed. I always ended up thanking God that I had thought to do whatever was needed—or had I? On at least two occasions that I can remember, I have awakened from a sound sleep with an idea about a case that, when tried in the morning either made the diagnosis or was helpful in the solution of the case.

I am certain these are acts of God.

Since Akron Children's Hospital was the designated center for all cases of polio—regardless of age—for eleven counties of Ohio, it is necessary for the reader to have some conception of how big a problem this was in the world. Referring to *The History of Polio* as published by: www.cloudnet.com/-curbsaass/poliotimeline.htm and accessed through Google under "Polio 1954," a timeline of the history of the disease is available. It was first described in the late 1700's, described in detail in the 1840's, and identified as caused by a virus in 1908. The first large outbreak in the U.S. was in 1916 when there were over 9,000 cases in New York City alone.

The polio virus attacked the anterior horn cells of the spinal cord—that part of the cord which empowers us to move, and once there, the damage was permanent; paralysis resulted. If the virus attacked the cranial nerves, this was called bulbar paralysis and was nearly always fatal.

In the 1930s when I was a child, there were severe outbreaks on the west coast and also on the east coast. There was a huge outbreak in my hometown. My parents took us to the shore of Connecticut to a cottage in Branford at Indian Neck on July first. We did not return until October, when Mom felt it was safe to do so. In New England, it was a summer time disease.

One of the worst years was 1952 when there were 58,000 cases in the U.S., and I had my first intimate encounter with the disease in my intern year when one of my boyhood friends was admitted to New Britain General Hospital complaining of being unable to breathe. A spinal tap was positive for polio, and he was put in an "iron lung." This was a tube into which the body of the patient was inserted from the neck down. It was a mechanical device which rhythmically decreased the pressure inside, making the lungs inflate (inhale) and then increased the pressure to make the lungs deflate (exhale). We transferred him to McCook Hospital in Hartford, which was Connecticut's contagious disease hospital. To get him there in his iron lung, we loaded him in the back of a pickup truck and I hand pumped the lung all the way, following a police escort to the McCook Hospital.

He died of a stress ulcer within two days.

In 1954, my first year at Akron Children's, we had over six hundred cases, of which twenty-five were grown men, and all the men died. They all had bulbar polio, which was almost always fatal, and involved the cranial nerves, especially the ones that make us breathe. The complete fatality in adult men was not as predictable in kids. I saw two or three completely recover from it.

There were about an equal number of adult women victims that summer. One of them delivered a baby while in an iron lung. At the time of the delivery she was taken out of the lung and received assisted breathing from an anesthesiologist. The delivery was otherwise uneventful, and both mother and child did well. Before leaving the hospital, the mother was almost totally well, and the baby was unscathed.

One early evening I had a ten-year-old youngster who came in complaining of headache, with a fever of 102. On physical exam he had two ominous signs: absent abdominal reflexes and a stiff neck. When we tried to flex his neck while he was lying on his back, he cried out in pain and came up with no flexion. Also, with him on his back, if I lifted his leg straight up without letting the knee bend, he had pain in his back. Because of these signs and symptoms, I was preparing to do a spinal tap on him.

"Tommy, I need to have you help me a little," I said to him, "We need to do a test on your back, and mostly it isn't going to hurt at all, except for a little prick at the beginning, when I am going to make your back go to sleep a little bit, so nothing will hurt you, okay?"

"Okay, doctor," he said bravely.

"Okay, fine. Now I would like you to lie on your left side—that's right. Now bring your knees up to your chin, and your chin down to your knees, like a little ball. That's great!"

Tommy was bent into a little ball with his knees and chin almost touching.

"Now, Tommy, in order to help you stay like that, Florence, my aide here, is going to put her left arm around your upper legs, and her right arm around your neck, okay?"

Florence had wrapped her left arm around his legs and her right around his neck, and had her hands locked together in the middle of the abdomen of the rolled up youngster. She placed her chin over his right hip to hold it down on the table.

"Okay, Tommy, this'll feel cold," I told him as I prepped the area. Then I draped him and was ready for the tap in a sterile field.

"Now this is the part that may hurt a little bit, but it will only be for a second or two, Tommy. You can swear if you want to."

Tommy giggled then said, "Ouch! Is that all?"

"That's all you should feel Tommy," I said.

Florence clamped down with her chin on Tommy's pelvic bone and pulled him together. The spinal needle went in easily, and just as easily I felt it pop into the canal.

But from the time Florence pulled him together, Tommy started objecting and then shouted, "Let me out! This is terrible! I can't stand it!" The more he struggled, the firmer was the pull by Florence, and the more snugly his face was in her armpit. He struggled and gasped and pleaded throughout the whole procedure and I couldn't understand why because there was no pain. We were just waiting for the spinal fluid to drip out for the three specimen tubes.

Finally we were done and Florence released her hold on a sweating red-faced little boy, who came up from under her arm gasping with relief. "That smell was terrible!" he panted, and as Florence, equally sweaty by this time wafted by, I understood immediately the source of Tommy's agony.

Happily, while Tommy's spinal fluid was positive for viral infection, which turned out not to be polio, but mumps. He had mumps encephalitis, and recovered without any problem.

That was the year that Salk vaccine came out, and in my second year (1955) I was there for polio time (summer), there were only one hundred to two hundred cases. This was the direct result of a tremendous effort to vaccinate all the kids before the season.

On one occasion I was assigned to vaccinate the children in a Catholic orphanage, and as I sat near the table with the supplies, two nuns would drag a screaming five- to nine-year old child up, and I would give him or/her the shot. This was always followed by, "God bless you, doctor," coming from a tear-stained face. Not one child forgot to bless me.

The analysis of the vaccination effort of 1954 showed clearly that it was successful, so a massive effort was made to vaccinate all the children, by 1957 there were only five thousand-plus cases in the United States. In 1964, one hundred twenty-one cases were reported.

The early 1990s saw huge efforts by China, India, and the UN to vaccinate against this dread disease. In those years, millions of youngsters were vaccinated in those countries.

There are still cases being reported from Africa, despite a UN resolution to have the disease wiped out by the year 2000.

At about 2:00 one morning, I received a call from the emergency room that there was a father down there with his five-month-old baby. He wanted someone right away, because his baby's foreskin was "stuck." In the uncircumcised newborn, pulling the foreskin back over the head of the penis could be quite a tight fit, and to the faint-hearted or ignorant person, it could appear to get stuck. I was annoyed to be gotten out of bed for such a stupid reason, so when I arrived at the room to fix this, I was less than cordial. The foreskin was clamped tightly around the crown of the glans, and the baby was crying loudly, as it must have hurt, so I asked the father, "How long has this been like this, and how did it get this way? Who pulled it back this far?"

"Doc, this is what I found when I went in to see why he was crying."

"Well, Mr. Gombatz, this didn't just happen. Somebody pulled the foreskin back that far and left it there."

"Are you suggesting that I did that, doctor?" he asked testily.

"Well, somebody did sir; who else is at your home besides you and your wife?"

At this point I put on some gloves, grasped the foreskin, and pulled it back to the front of the penis. The baby stopped crying right away." I don't like your attitude, doctor. You are being rude, and I am going to report you to the administrator in the morning!" blustered Mr. Gombatz.

""You do that, Mr. Gombatz, and while you are at it, explain to the administrator what you were doing playing with your son's penis at two in the morning!" I took off the gloves, threw them in the waste basket, and stomped out of the room.

There was never a complaint registered.

Just at the end of the first year, Dr. Kramer, who was the chief of staff, and in fact the reason that there was a Children's Hospital in Akron, called me aside one day.

"Rackliffe, I want you to be chief resident this next year. What do you think?"

"Gosh! Dr. Kramer, I don't really feel qualified to take that job."

"Well, I think you are, and you have had an extra year of training that none of the others have had, so you are my choice."

I was stunned, but I replied, "All right sir, and thank you for the vote of confidence." I couldn't have been more proud! This man was a god to me, and to have him trust me was a real feather in my cap. Besides, it came with a raise and a nice house right next to the parking lot of the hospital.

Dr. Kramer then continued, "At Children's Hospital as chief resident, you are responsible for every patient in the hospital, regardless of whose service they are on. All the attending staff knows that you have the power to countermand any order, but you had better be right if you do such a thing." He smiled, but there was no smile in his voice, this was putting me on notice, and I determined to make hospital rounds every day with the surgical and orthopedic residents, as well as with the medical ones.

I couldn't wait to see Jane's face when I told her about it, especially since we were expecting again, and the extra room and nice house would be great.

I soon learned that the "buck stops here." Within a month, one of my senior residents came to me.

"Bob, would you be really unhappy if I asked you to release me from my contract? I've been thinking it over, and I really don't like pediatrics. I like the children all right, but the mothers drive me crazy."

Boy! This was familiar ground for me, and my answer was right on the table in a flash. "Roy, if you are not happy here, the time to leave is now. By all means, get yourself set up in what you want, and good luck to you."

"It's great of you to let me go, and I appreciate it."

"I wouldn't have it any other way, and good luck."

(That's the way it should be done, Dr. Snowman!)

The buck stopping at my door also meant that if there was a procedure needing to be done and none of the other residents could do it (which was rare), I was called to decide what to do, or do it myself.

The toughest job I got in my year as chief resident was doing an exchange transfusion on a three-pound premie that had been shipped in from a small hospital down state. His umbilical vein (which is the vein always used) had been traumatized by the local doctors, to the point that it was useless for an exchange. So I did the exchange using his right Radial artery, just above the wrist, to get the blood out and a scalp vein to replace the blood I took out. I exchanged three hundred ccs (which is just a tad more than half a unit of blood), and I thought that was enough for this size "premie. He did very well, and when he had gained the requisite five pounds, we sent him home with his anxious, but happy parents.

In 1956, there was no measles vaccine, and his disease was with us every year, and was vicious. Characterized by symptoms such as a cold for the first day or so, followed by a fever up to 104–106, these symptoms could last as long as a week. It was a serious disease. The rash would start to show about the third day of fever and start on the head, going down to the legs as the fever finally subsided. There were all sorts of complications from it; convulsions from the high fever, pneumonia, and encephalitis (inflammation of the brain caused by the measles virus), and even death.

One of the ways to assure a slight case without any problems was to deliberately expose a child to the disease, followed one week later by giving the child an injection of Gamma globulin, which had antibodies to the disease in it. This would reduce the severity of the disease. It was a common practice and was usually successful.

Roger, age ten, was adopted, and the only child of the Morans. During the measles outbreak that year their pediatrician had recommended he be exposed, and then one week later be given an injection of gamma globulin to make the illness less serious.

In Roger's case, it didn't work. When he came down with the measles, his temperature shot up to 106 and stayed there.

He was admitted to the hospital and a spinal tap was done. The cerebral spinal fluid showed presence of white cells, signifying encephalitis. There was nothing to do but keep him well hydrated and try to keep the temperature down.

Despite heroic efforts and constant care, Roger died on the fourth day of his admission.

From that day on, I never, ever advocated exposing a child to anything deliberately. Such planned exposures to disease were frequently done, especially with chicken pox, even more often than measles, and in my fifty years of practice, I saw children die from all the "harmless" childhood diseases: mumps, chicken pox, and many from measles.

We had pretty much settled in to a nice routine at Children's, and my surgical and orthopedic residents were a pleasure to work with. Most of the staff got along pretty well with the house staff, except for one pediatrician that really got my attention the first year I was there. On New Year's Eve, there was a flurry of admissions of his kids with a diagnosis of "pneumonia." None of them looked sick, and indeed, most were discharged New Year's Day. All of these admissions came from the office of one pediatrician, Dr. Panda.

He was using the hospital to supply baby sitting for these kids. I mentioned it to the chief of staff and the next year when it started again on New Year's Eve day, I called the Dr. Kramer right away.

"Dr. Kramer, this is Bob Rackliffe, and I am sorry to bother you sir, but Dr. Panda has admitted six kids today with diagnoses of pneumonia, and none of them is coughing, none has a fever, and he hasn't even ordered chest x-rays. This is exactly what he did last year, too, sir, and I think we are just being used for baby sitting."

"Are you sure that none of them is sick?" he asked.

"Yes sir."

"Alright. What is his office number? I will speak to him."

I gave him the number of Dr. Panda's private line.

About twenty minutes later, Dr. Panda called and discharged all six patients.

From that point on, Dr. Panda was understandably quiet around me.

In January 1956, our fourth son was born, and he was a beauty! A big and handsome baby, he was born at Akron General Hospital. The news traveled quickly cross town to Children's, and Myrt, the telephone operator at the hospital, announced it over the public address paging system. "Attention please! Dr. and Mrs. Rackliffe had their fourth baby boy this morning. Both mother and child are doing well." There was a collective groan throughout the hospital, since many were rooting for a girl. For our part, we were delighted to add the fourth and final member of our family: Steven Lockwood Rackliffe (Lockwood was my maternal great grandmother's maiden name).

We both loved the trusting, straight out, "tell it like it is" attitude that separates the mind of a boy from that of a girl.

My chief surgical resident, Charlie was a prince of a guy with an awkward last name: Fuchs. This was pronounced phonetically: *fewks*. The trouble was that a lot of people didn't pronounce it phonetically. Charlie and I got to be great friends, and while he was at Children's, he developed a relationship with a simply great girl "Precie" Seiberling, who volunteered full time at Children's. Jane and I enjoyed their company and were delighted to hear they were engaged, and also pleased to hear that Charlie, with perhaps a little urging form Precie, had his named changed to Fox.

Much better.

As the time came to get ready to leave Children's, Dr. Kramer asked me what I would like as a gift from him and the staff.

"I know that all of my senior residents and I would like a picture of you, sir."

He complied with our wishes and was very pleased at the engraved gold cuff links we had made for him.

What a great human being.

When the time came to say good bye to my senior residents, to the staff at the hospital, and to those residents who were becoming the new senior residents, Jane and I were filled with emotion as we started to pack and prepare to come back to New Britain to open an office for the practice of pediatrics and settle down for the rest of our lives. The years since our marriage had been challenging and fun, our four little boys were the icing on the cake, and now finally, we were going home to do what George Radford and I had pledged in the jungle of Saipan: To serve God by serving our fellow man.

PART 8

OPENING PRACTICE

We started for New Britain, Connecticut, from Akron, Ohio, at night and planned to drive all night from Akron. That way, the boys would sleep most of the way home. The plan worked out well, and the trip was uneventful except for the Pennsylvania Turnpike. On that speedway, we were surrounded by trucks going at frightening speeds. There were huge numbers of dead deer lying along the road from one end of it to the other. It was a sad sight. I was glad that the boys were asleep, as there were so many of those beautiful animals slaughtered by the cars and trucks that it was heartbreaking, as well as worrisome; suppose one darted out in front of us?

Jane and I shared driving as we often did on trips: two hours on and two hours off was the plan, and it helped to keep us alert. Our departure time from Akron was such that we arrived in Connecticut at around 8:00 a.m.

All the boys were awake by 6:00 a.m., and the "Are we there yets?" as well as the bathroom stops started about 6:15 and were immediately addressed. We pulled off the road for breakfast at one of the service stations situated on the turnpike, and then resumed our homeward trek. There was increasing anticipation for all of us as we drew closer to what was to be our home, with the boys getting more excited by the mile. They burst into shouts of joy when we rounded the curve and could see Nana and Buck's 1890 house on the next corner, welcoming us. It stood there: a big, square three-story house with a porch all across the front of what had initially been a duplex, changed into a single home by my grandfather.

In the front yard, as if to emphasize the dominance of the huge house, was an oak tree with a trunk that was seven feet in diameter, its branches reaching out to protect the three-story home in concert with an ancient maple, which guarded the driveway and the northern part of the house. Between them was the slate walk to the porch and entrance.

The fifteen room house owned that corner and frowned at the smaller houses across the street. It was in a corner of the remaining fifteen acres of what had been a fifty-acre farm at one time. There was a typical Yankee red barn in the back yard with a ramp across the entire barn which led to three garages and raised hay trucks up to the hay door on the second floor.

The second floor windows of the house overlooking the driveway were in the room where I had been born, and my father before me.

As we drove down the gravel driveway, the stones made crunching noises that sounded so familiar and so welcoming. We parked under the sickle pear tree, as Mom and Dad came down the steps to greet us, hugging and kissing each boy and taking turns holding Stevie whom they were seeing and holding for the first time.

Jane's dad had told us that the house being built for us on Lewis Road had just had the cellar poured the week before we left Akron, so that meant that we would be living with my folks in the old homestead for a considerable length of time.

"No problem!" said my dad. "You pay the food bill and we'll take care of the rest." Well, the food bill and the way my mother ordered food was an eye opener to Jane.

Lunches and dinners were formal; i.e., table cloths, napkins (linen), and two or three course meals at dinner. Lunch was always something warm; e.g., soup plus sandwiches or salads, or both.

Dinner always started with a fruit cup, followed by the main course, which was some kind of meat that my dad would carve at the table while he was carrying on with the boys. When Jimmy asked him to pass the rolls, he threw one to him, which started an epidemic of flying rolls and lots of laughter. Love and happiness were a constant in my folks' home.

It was expected that after dinner each night as dessert was being served, Dad would select a symphony or concerto from his collection, and we would all sit at the dining room table and listen to it in its entirety.

His favorite composer was Rachmaninoff, and he passed his love of music on to all of his children. The boys immediately got the message, although "Buck," as all the grandchildren called him, cut the length of his selections because of their age.

The boys were fascinated by the house, so we explored it together. There were two front doors, because it had been a duplex when my grandfather bought it. Each doorway had a stained-glass window. The one on the right that was off the library had been converted to a lavatory. The stairway to the second floor was double width because of the conversion from a duplex to a single home. At the bottom of the stairway it opened to the dining room on the left and the library on the right. The library was dad's favorite room. All the chairs were red leather, one with a hassock, and there was a floor-to-ceiling bookcase along the entire inner wall.

A huge console, which was the source of the music, occupied one wall, along with a huge number of records all in shelving. The music, usually classical, was piped throughout the house on every floor, via multiple strategically placed speakers on all three floors. On the walls in all the rooms there were gas lamps that were still functional. A huge cherry tree that was taller than the house stood outside the library windows.

All across the front of the house was the living room, which entered both the dining room on the left and the library on the right.

Going to the back of the house through either the library or the dining room, one came to a vast room that spanned the width of the house, serving as a modern kitchen on the dining room side and a casual dining area on the library side. Both sides of the kitchen opened onto porches that led to back stairs. The porch on the library side was a sun porch with wicker furniture.

The porch on the kitchen side was for rubbish, garbage cans, and, from a side window, a clothesline ran from the house to a tree in the woods, where a pulley like the one on the porch allowed the hanging of clothes all the way from the house into the woods, across the driveway at a height of thirty-five feet.

The boys had as much fun in the old barn as I had had when I was a child. There were all kinds of secret places to investigate, and to their delight, it was full of trap doors and hiding places; perfect for "cowboys and Indians." The barn had housed a cow, pigs, and chickens during World War II, but throughout my early life, it had been used just as a three-car garage and for storage of windows, window frames, and oak molding from the company. There were also a lot of agricultural things in there, such as silage pipe, plow parts, and even some metal seats for tractors. To get all this stuff in the second-floor space for hay, they backed the trucks up the ramp to the door originally used to offload hay. At that level, it was a cinch to store the bulky or heavy equipment.

Jimmy was intrigued by the pipes and chains on the walls of the different rooms in the house. He didn't see any in the barn, so when we returned to the house, he pointed at one and said, "What are those things, Dad?" as he pointed to the gas lamps.

"Those are gas lights, Jim. When this house was built, there wasn't any electricity, and Gommie and Gompie had gaslight." (Gommie and Gompie were Dad's parents, and the names were given to them by my sister when she was a little tot).

"In 1938 we had a hurricane here that knocked down eleven big trees in Gommie and Gompie's yard, and we were without electricity for over a week, so Gompie brought home mantles (just like the kind in our Coleman lantern), and tied them on the pipes and then lit them. The little chain controls the amount of gas being used. We used them for over a week and were glad they were here."

Then I continued. "They closed school for a week or so, and Buck and Gompie brought home some axes and a six-foot, two-man saw, a couple of Buck saws, and we cut those eleven trees up and rolled them down the hill towards Willow Brook, where they lay until they rotted away."

By this time we were about to go up to the third floor, and I thought I would tell the boys about the big mystery in the house.

"You boys keep a sharp lookout in all the places you explore, because Buck thinks that Gompie might have hidden $75,000 somewhere in here. You'll see Buck every now and then digging up the earthen cellar floor, or checking for loose bricks; he's always looking for the money."

By this time we were in one of the two bedrooms on the third floor with a bathroom in between them. In the bathroom there was another gas light, a claw-foot tub, and a toilet with a chain you pulled to make it flush. I pointed to a part of the wall between the tub and toilet that had a covered opening in it.

"Look at that, boys. Wonder where that goes?"

"Can we go in there, Dad, and see?" questioned Jimmy, with Danny nodding vigorously.

"Sure," I said, "I think there is a flashlight in this closet." I found it and handed it to Jimmy. "Go ahead, Jim, see what's in there."

He hesitated. "You coming, too?" he asked tentatively.

"Right behind you, son."

He and Dan pulled out the obstructing panel and looked into a fourteen-foot dark space right under the roof.

They cautiously crept through the hole and into the space. There was nothing in there except floor boards, which they checked to see if any were loose.

"Looks empty to me," said Danny, "let's get out of here." Jimmy and Peter were quick to agree.

Finally, we got to the storage area of the house, which was the entire front half of the third floor.

There was a window in the center of the front wall that helped to illuminate a room full of trunks, suitcases, and garment bags (one of them had my Air Force uniforms in it), but the boys didn't find any money there either.

That money had been a cash payment to my grandfather, who sold the sash and door part of his business to another man in town. Even now that business is flourishing and is still owned by the same family that originally bought it from my grandfather.

Dad wanted to find that money. He knew that it had never been banked or shown up on the company ledgers, and while he hoped and kept looking, he suspected that my grandfather had given it to a woman in another town with whom he was having an affair.

Gompie used to go one day a week by streetcar to the town where she lived, which must have taken a while, because he had to change trolleys in Hartford to go north to her town. I think by the time we kids were on the scene, that affair was history, but when that house comes down, there may be a surprise for some lucky person.

In the early 1990s when I was the school physician, I told an especially disruptive high school student who was living in that house that there was $75,000 hidden in there somewhere. I bet that turned a few bricks over. It might have lifted a few attic floorboards, too.

The next day I showed the boys the grove and told them the stories about how my grandfather had always enjoyed working around the fifteen acres and had planted a flower garden next to the barn where the chicken coop had been, with stone walls front and back and a wire fence along the length of it. Then he had made a lawn from the back of the barn for about one hundred fifty to two hundred yards through some fruit trees to a little goldfish pond that he had made. He connected the fountain in the pool to the well under the back steps of the house. Beyond the goldfish pool alongside a grove of oaks, there was a professional croquet court and a clay tennis court. There was an outhouse discretely placed on the gravelly road that led down past the barn to "The Grove."

On the right side of the lawn leading to the grove was a lot about five hundred feet by five hundred feet that he used for vegetables. At the edge of that piece, there were eight to ten apple trees bordering his property line.

The grove was a special place. There were two woven hammocks suspended between large oak trees, plenty of parking space, and in the center of the grove of oak trees, there was a pavilion about forty-five feet long by thirty feet wide, replete with a floor and two long tables of about sixteen feet each, beautifully made, with matching benches.

Right alongside the pavilion on an outcropping of flat rock, there was a brick fireplace. It was complete with an iron pipe grill and warming area, and played an important part of each weekend.

To the south of the grove was a professionally maintained croquet ground with half-inch thick iron wickets, all painted white, on a lawn made of creeping bent grass (like the greens on a golf course) that was mowed short and rolled every week.

The same roller was used to keep the clay tennis court that adjoined the croquet ground smooth and hard.

South of the croquet ground and to the border of the property was swampland with a couple of springs running from it into Willow Brook Park, which it adjoined on the east border. When I was growing up, there were plans to dig out that swamp and make it into a swimming pool, but the Depression pushed that off until it was too late.

The grove was an ideal place for three young boys to play, and on Sundays it was full of family and friends. Every family brought food and drink to share. Croquet and tennis games went on all day long.

Later, when my grandmother's arthritis got too bad for her to walk, my grandfather bought a balloon-tired wheel barrow and would wheel her, sitting on the front edge and hanging on to the sides, laughing and bouncing all the way to the grove.

Seeing that tennis court reminded me of the time, when at age thirteen, I first beat my grandfather. He always played with his shirt buttoned and his winged collar and tie in place. As we were walking off the court, he said with a tear in his eye, "Well, Bobbie, you finally beat me."

I felt terrible.

Ever since the Depression in the 1930s, the grove had been a gathering place on spring, summer, and fall Sundays for neighbors, friends, and friends of friends to gather and play tennis and croquet all day long.

The courts were never empty, and the competition was fierce on both playing fields, occasionally riling up tempers on the croquet grounds when someone was being mauled by an opponent.

No one had any money, so when they needed a new tennis net, it took ten men to get $35 together for a new net.

People usually started arriving between eight and nine, and the last ones would leave after supper at night as the light failed. Everyone would bring something to eat such as casseroles, potato salad, baked beans, home made pies (which will never be forgotten), and brownies.

My grandmother "Gommie" would make her famous coffee in an old huge grey enamel coffee pot (about twenty-five cup size) by bringing the water to a boil, then throwing in the coffee tied in cheesecloth, putting on the lid, then letting it steep after setting the pot on the warming area of the brick fireplace

"There has never been a better coffee made than that," Dad said emphatically.

On the fireplace, my dad would be cooking hamburgers, hot dogs, and toasting buns over a bed of glowing charcoal. When all was ready, twenty-five to thirty people would seat themselves around the two picnic tables my grandfather had had made, and the meal would begin with a lot of taunting of the losers and much good fun and joviality.

It was the midst of the Depression, but you wouldn't have known it in that loving and heartwarming little bit of heaven.

On the first day of work as a practicing physician, I entered my half of our new office where there was a nice desk and chair—a gift from Harold, my senior partner. Then I looked at the tables that the carpenter at my father's business had made to the specifications I had taken of the tables in the ER at Children's Hospital. Perfect! They were as high as the ones there so that there was very little bending required. I laughed out loud at the look of them—great!

The drawers at the head of the table slid in and out with ease and were all the right sizes for stethoscope, diagnostic set, surgical instruments, and prescription pads.

From the stack of drawers about a foot off the floor at one end of the table, there was an empty shelf extending to the end of the table. The table tops were padded with vinyl and cushioning.

I stood against the table and practiced bending down to an imaginary baby.

Perfect!

Harold introduced me to his nurse of twenty-odd years, Mrs. Ahearn. She said, "Good to see you finally after all this planning, doctor. It seems like it took forever."

"Hi, Mrs. Ahearn. Good to see you again. It sure did seem like forever to us, too."

Harold had arranged to have my office phone number put in the new telephone book, and I quickly arranged to have my office number put in the bedroom we were using at the folks' home.

For $200, the phone company ran a line down to the grove with a jack there for use when I was down there. (This was like a long leash, for there were no beepers or cell phones in those days. With a phone in the grove it made life easier and happier since I could spend more time with the family.)

Harold had arranged for a few patients to see me the first day. I did okay with that, but they were his patients, and we were all aware of that, so I felt uncomfortable and tolerated under the very watchful eye of the mothers.

It is a customary courtesy for any new physician to call on the other doctors in town and introduce himself, and also to send out announcements of his opening a practice. So for several afternoons, I was busy introducing myself to the other pediatricians, aand the obstetricians, and the few general practice men in town.

My first very own patient came as a referral from an obstetrician in Bristol, who happened to be a McGill graduate. He sent me a new young couple with their first baby, and it was love at first sight!

Ruthie Cavanaugh was just a sweet person with a throaty soft chuckle, and when she came in, she shook my hand, and with a big warm smile said, "Dr. Rackliffe, my obstetrician is Dr. Purney in Bristol, and he recommended you very highly."

"Well, Mrs. Cavanaugh, I'm pleased to hear that. I have never met Dr. Purney, but I have heard nothing but good things about him."

We hit it off immediately, and I became quite friendly with her and her husband, who was a real funny guy; he always had a witty saying and a ready laugh. In later years I played golf against him in a tournament, and he showed up on the first tee in a tuxedo, including the shiny shoes!

Ruthie and John ended up with five children, and they were adorable little Irish cherubs with a mischievous gleam in their eyes almost always. Whenever they came into the office as a family, I was impressed at how loving and concerned these children were for their siblings and how great the relationship was with the parents.

The first night I was on call, we had finished dinner and were all sitting around in the living room, watching an eight-inch TV (the usual boxing show) and waiting for the phone to ring. I was on pins and needles; I hoped that it wasn't someone with a problem that I wouldn't be able to treat. There was not much talking, everyone was just waiting. When the phone did ring, everyone cheered! It was a new mother whose baby wouldn't stop crying, so she wanted me to come out.

"Does he have a fever?"

"I don't know; I don't know how to take his temperature."

"Okay, Mrs. Newjewski, I will be right out."

As she hung up the phone, I heard her say, "It's Dr. Greenblatt's assistant and he is coming out."

I found her house on the other side of town and went up to their second floor apartment and was welcomed. There was a cake of soap and towel by the kitchen sink, and the baby who had been crying and when I got there was still putting up a fuss and acting starved.

"Could I see the bottle please?" I asked after assuring myself that the baby was not sick, just hungry.

The mother handed me the bottle, which had only the three holes in the nipple made by the manufacturer.

"I think I need a small sewing needle and a pair of pliers, please."

When this was supplied, I went over to the gas stove and lit a burner, and holding the needle with the pliers, I put it in the flame until it was white hot and then quickly pierced the nipple with it. I repeated this several more times so that the milk flowed easily.

Then I said, "Mrs. Newjewski, please get another diaper and then sit down here with me."

She complied.

When she was seated, I wrapped the diaper around the child's neck, bunched up behind his head and seated him upright on her left thigh.

"Now Mrs. Newjewski, sit the baby just as he is in this upright position with your left hand supporting his head and give him the bottle with the nipple just full of milk but without the weight of the milk on the nipple."

Once in his mouth that little guy started taking it as fast as he could with very little effort.

"Oh my, doctor! He's taking it so fast! Shouldn't I stop to burp him?"

"No. He'll stop in a minute or so when he is ready to burp. You just sit there with him upright and he will burp himself."

Directly after saying that, it happened as predicted; he stopped, sat there for a moment, and then produced a huge dry burp.

Within fifteen minutes, the bottle was empty and the baby was asleep.

"Well thank you so very much for coming, doctor. I think I get the idea now," said Mrs. Newjewski as she stood with her pocket book in hand at the door.

"That'll be $5 please."

With that, I called in, and since there were no more calls, I headed for home!

That was kind of neat! I felt really pleased at the way that had gone.

Back in 1956, pediatricians made house calls. In fact the patients' parents would call and order a house call by the doctor on call as if they were ordering a loaf of bread. Ten to fifteen house calls per day were not out of the ordinary. I didn't like the fact that the decision to make a house call was being made by a non-medical person and was afraid that someone who really needed to be seen would be put off because of calls that were not necessary. After all, you could only do as many as time would allow, so a decision as to whether or not a house call was needed was a constant source of worry.

I recall being ordered to the house of Mr. Beach, a very important executive of one of the large local manufacturing companies one evening. His children were patients of Harold's. After examining the child I said, "This is just a little cold, probably viral. Just keep him in for a day or two and give him aspirin or Tylenol if he is uncomfortable. Please call us if anything like a sore throat or ear ache occurs, and we will take care of it, but I am very reassured after seeing him that he'll be fine."

Mr. Beach said, "I want you to give him a shot of penicillin."

"That isn't necessary in this case, sir, and could be dangerous. There can be undesirable side effects."

"Nevertheless I want you to give him a shot."

I couldn't believe my ears.

"How much would you like him to have, and what kind?" I asked him, curious to see what he would say.

He stepped right into it! "I don't know- you're the doctor."

"Well now that we have established that fact, I think a shot is not indicated, and I repeat my instructions to you to call if there is any change that concerns you."

I closed my bag, washed my hands, all the while sensing the anger in the room.

The next morning, Harold was called to the house to see the child. I don't know whether the child got penicillin or not, but from then on, when they needed a doctor, Harold would go, whether on call or not. I never saw the children of that family again.

When I started in practice with Harold, mornings were reserved for hospital visits and house calls, and we had office hours afternoons only and then more house calls at night. There were times when I would be driving ten miles to Southington, and pass Harold coming back from there, which never failed to strike me as stupid and wasteful.

Still, house calls could be fun. Whenever I had to go to the Barrows house, I knew there would be a fresh baked chocolate cream pie, cooling on the kitchen table with a plate, fork, and napkin waiting nearby.

There was an Italian family who ran a bakery right next to their house, and a house call there was guaranteed to produce a still warm crusty loaf of Italian bread. This happened once on a Sunday, so when I finished the house call I called Jane in the middle of house calls, to tell her of the welcome gift I would be bringing home. Jane made pasta with meat balls, and when I got home, we devoured that whole loaf, still warm, along with the pasta. yum! Was it good!

I had another family in Berlin with five or six children. One time I made a house call there, and Kathy (the mom) gave me a basket of tomatoes for the visit. That was fine with me; it wasn't taxable and tasted great.

Over the years, I developed some absolutely delightful relationships with some of my mothers. One playfully disrespectful Irish mom was just so much fun. Whenever she was in the office, my nurse would come in to me laughing, and tell me that Maureen Connolly said, "to get my ragged ass in gear, she had a hair appointment." So when it was time for her to be brought in to a room, I would go to the door and call, "Okay, you old bat, come on in and let's get it over with!" Both of us enjoyed the banter, and the expressions on the faces of the other people in the waiting room were priceless, but soon changed from shock to smiles at the ongoing ribbing.

As she got up to come into the examining rooms she would start again. "It's about time! If you knew what you were doing, it wouldn't take so long; come on, Carol, let's go see if he can do something right!" This conversation was always at about forty decibels, so that everyone in the office could hear it, which invariably led to laughter. Oh, she was fun! Every one of us in the office enjoyed her visits and repartee.

One afternoon, I completed my office hours earlier than my partner Harold, and he asked me to make a house call for him because the baby really sounded in pain and I could get there quicker than he could. So I threw my bag in the car and went to the baby's home. As I got out of the car, I could hear a baby screaming in a third floor apartment. The mother was waiting when I climbed the stairs to her kitchen door. She stood there rocking the inconsolable baby back and forth. Tears streamed down her face.

"Let's put the baby on the bed, Mrs. Bonola, so I can examine him."

She laid him down. He continued to scream and kick. His face was red and covered with sweat. He was in constant motion, kicking and screaming.

"When did he start to cry?" I asked.

"When I got him up from his nap," she replied.

At that point, I started to take off his shoes and undress him, as I had been taught to do in Med School: Take off all the clothes before the exam.

As I untied the shoes I noticed that the instep was much higher on the right shoe than the instep of the left shoe and as I removed the right shoe, I could see that the baby's forefoot had been bent back under the rear part of the foot. As the foot came out of the shoe and unfolded, the baby shuddered and gave a deep gasp, stopped crying, and in a heart beat, was fast asleep.

Mrs. Bonola had inadvertently bent the forefoot back on itself when she put the shoe on, causing unimaginably intense pain for the little guy.

Another case comes to mind at once. A friend who was a physician called me one morning and asked if I would see his eleven-year-old son, Ken. The boy had been complaining of a stomachache the entire weekend. Another physician, a surgeon, and neighbor of his, had looked at him, and neither one of them could make a diagnosis.

Of course, I agreed to see him immediately.

"Great, Bob, my wife will bring him in. Please call me at the office after you have seen him."

She arrived in less than a half hour. My nurse showed him in to one of the examining rooms, and told him to take off everything but his underpants.

When I entered the room, it was immediately apparent that Ken was in considerable discomfort. There was a look of pain and apprehension on his face. His movements were very slow and careful as if it hurt to move. He looked gray.

"I think I'm going to throw up," he said.

As I felt his abdomen, it was painful for him. I lifted up his body and pulled down his briefs, so that the whole abdomen would be visible, and there was a huge inguinal hernia on the right side!

Inguinal hernias occur when the intestines go through the inguinal canal into the scrotum in males (or much less frequently the labia in females).

The inguinal canal is a hole shaped like a tube running right through the abdominal muscles that allows the veins, arteries, vas and testicle to connect to the urethra at the level of the prostate.

In the fetus the testicle, which starts life on the back wall of the abdomen, is literally pulled down and out through the abdominal wall to the scrotum.

In my friend's son's case, the hernia was huge, and I could feel loops of small intestine in the scrotum.

When I called his father to tell him what his son's problem was, there was silence on the line for a period of time, but then his response was exactly what mine would have been in similar circumstances. "Shit!"

I understood how he felt. He had missed something, and so had his friend by simply not being thorough. If they had removed the clothes, the diagnosis would have been made, and he would have been cured by simple surgery. He must have felt like an idiot.

At any rate, the surgeon operated on Ken, and he did very well. I'm sure everyone involved in the case learned a lesson (including me): "You are not examining clothes, you are examining a person; take all the clothes off!"

When I first opened my office, the waiting room was comfortable, with sofas and some overstuffed chairs and looked like a living room to make it homelike with pictures and a painting on the walls.

We played classical music during office hours, which had a very positive effect on keeping noise and behavior at a much nicer level; it was piped through the office as background music during the whole day and commented on favorably by many of the parents.

By September our house was finished, and we moved into our own home for the first time. It was a Cape Cod with two bedrooms and a bath upstairs, and a bedroom, dining room, living room, bath, and a spacious kitchen downstairs. We were delighted. It was in a new housing project and most all of the owners were our age.

Children were abundant. Dad Baldwin had picked out the best lot on the street, very big and flat; great for the kids to run around in and very safe because the roads were full of curves and served only the development.

One night after dinner, when I signed in with the answering service, there were seven house calls plus eight or nine phone calls. My circuit would create a big circular route that included a suburb. When I finally got to the last call around 10:00 p.m., I was met at the door by an anxious mother who quickly showed me into the room, where I examined a fussy baby who had no fever and was simply teething. Everything else was fine. I told the mother what the problem was and suggested she rub some medication for teething on the baby's gums and give the baby 0.8ml of Tylenol.

She paid me, and as I put on my coat and started toward the door she said, "Oh by the way doctor, your service called and said to tell you to call home because you have an emergency."

I could have killed her!

I called at once, and Jane answered the phone. "Oh, I am so glad you finally called! Peter says he swallowed a battery. He was acting kind of funny, and I asked what happened, and he said he choked on a battery, and then swallowed it."

"A battery? How big?"

"He showed me one like it, and it is about one half inch in diameter and an inch long. There is no paper or wrapping on it. I called my father, and he thought I should call you right away because the casing might be lead and he thought that might be dangerous."

"That is dangerous. I'll be right home, and I will be taking him up to the hospital for an x-ray."

Within a half hour I had asked another pediatrician to cover me, and I had ten-year-old Peter in the car on the way to the E.R. When I got there and ordered the x-ray, I spotted my boyhood friend and my favorite surgeon George Bray and asked him to stay around for a minute after telling him what had happened.

Sure enough, there on the x-ray of his stomach was a battery of about one inch in length, just like the other lead-cased one at home.

Would letting it pass normally give him lead poisoning? Should we go in now and get it out?

"What do you think, Bob?" asked George. "If there is any doubt I can just go in and take it out right now. If it is not dangerous though, that would be an unnecessary risk."

"I don't know, George. I think I'll call down to Yale and ask them."

I put in a call to the pediatrician on call at Yale and hit the jackpot. He was playing poker with a group of physicians at one of their homes. My phone call was patched through. "Hi, Dr. Gibbs. This is Bob Rackliffe, a pediatrician in New Britain, and I need some advice, please."

"Yes, doctor, what can I do for you?"

"Well sir, I have a ten-year-old boy in the E.R. here with a one inch long lead-cased battery in his stomach and my question is, do we let it pass without danger of lead poisoning or do we take it out?"

"Hmm. Interesting, just a minute, doctor." I heard him present the problem to the group of physicians, then a lot of voices all going at once and finally:

"Doctor? The consensus here is that we think you can let it pass without any risk, but it is an interesting case. Let me know how it turns out."

"Thank you for your time and advice, doctor."

I turned to George. "They think it'll be all right, but they obviously didn't know for sure. What do you think?"

"It's easy enough to take out, Bob."

"Let's take it out tonight then, George and let's get a blood lead level now and in the morning to see what happens to it."

Before he went to surgery, the blood lead level was done and was three times the toxic level. The results of that blood test came back when Peter was in the recovery room and the battery was out. By 11:30 p.m., Peter was in bed sleeping on the pediatric floor, and Mommy was right there at his side. I signed back in, but luckily there were no calls, and Jane and I finally went home around 2 after Jane had reassured Peter she would be back in the morning.

In the morning, Peter was awake, well, and hungry. His blood lead level drawn at that time was back to normal.

In the morning I put in a call to Dr. Gibbs. "Dr. Gibbs? Bob Rackliffe here. I just wanted to report to you on the little boy with the battery in his stomach."

"Oh yes, doctor, how is he doing?"

"Well we did a blood lead level last night and it was three times the toxic level, so we removed it last night, and this morning's level is within normal limits."

"Interesting. Thanks for letting me know, doctor."

Some time later in the year, the chief of pediatrics, Dr. Johnson, paid me the highest of compliments. He asked me to consult on a patient he had just seen on a house call and was admitting him to the hospital. He was out making other house calls, but he was worried about this case, so he was happy to hear that I was still at the hospital. The baby boy was about a two- or three-month-old infant. He was comatose and did not respond even to painful stimuli. His pupils were dilated and did not react to light; an ominous sign. There was a large bruise about the size of a nickel on the left cheek and a hemorrhagic stripe next to the bruise. This told me all I needed to know. When a person is struck hard with an open hand, there will be linear hemorrhages corresponding to the spaces between the fingers). It was clearly a slap by a hand with a ring on the finger next to the pinkie.

After checking him all over, I looked in his eyes with an ophthalmoscope and saw fresh hemorrhages on the retina of each eye. These telltale signs told me that there had to be hemorrhages in the brain, too.

I called Dr. Johnson and said, "Ros, this boy has been beaten, and is brain-damaged, and probably will die in a short time. Do you want me to say anything to the mother?"

"That was what I thought, too, Bob. Don't say anything yet, I'm on my way up there now and I would prefer it if we saw her together."

"Okay, Ros."

Breathing became shallower, and as time ticked by, the beautiful little body struggled less and less, as if glad to leave such a terrible world. He died about fifteen minutes after Ros got there, and Ros and I went to the mother with the bad news she seemed to know was coming.

Dr. Johnson then reported the case to the hospital administrator as per hospital protocol, and the administrator notified the police. The mother's boyfriend, who was with her at the hospital, was charged with the murder.

I noticed he had a huge ring on his right fourth finger.

One of the great comforts of practicing in my area was the presence of excellent specialists available in almost every specialty.

One Sunday, one of my personal friends called me at home to say that her son had the croup so bad that he was having a hard time breathing. I went right over to see Tommy, a cute little Irish freckle-faced, blue-eyed boy. I walked in to hear him inhale from the hallway, and his bark-like cough sounded as though it must hurt terribly. He was having great difficulty breathing. He had a very severe case of the croup.

Croup is usually from a virus. It runs in families, and is much more common in spring and fall; i.e. with the change in seasons. It almost always starts at midnight or thereabouts. It is caused by swelling of the larynx and or trachea and bronchi, which causes obstruction of the airway. It is frightening to the child because he wakes up unable to breathe, and the sight frightens most parents, too. The usual case will improve on the way to the hospital because of the cold night air, which seems to soothe them.

This was not the case with Tommy. He was in desperate circumstances and working hard to get any air.

Immediately I put in a call from Tommy's home to the chief of ear, nose, and throat, Dr. Daley.

"I'll meet you at the hospital, Bob," was the reassuring reply.

We drove to the hospital in my VW Beetle, with Tommy's mom holding him.

When we arrived at the ER, the nurse waved us through to the surgical suite.

"Dr. Daley wants you to come straight down to surgery; he is already scrubbing." So Mom and I literally ran down to the surgical unit. I asked Mom to wait in the waiting room outside surgery, reassured her he would be okay, and carried Tom into the operating room.

After assessing Tommy's condition, Dr. Daley said, "We can't wait for an anesthesiologist; we have to go."

Tommy was barely alive and an awful blue color.

I stood very close to Tommy's ear and told him, "This is going to hurt for a minute, Tommy, but then you will feel great. Just be brave and hold my hand; it will be over soon." He nodded and lay still like a champion while Dr. Daley made an incision in his skin overlying the trachea, and then into the trachea itself, and deftly slipped the cannula into the trachea in one motion. Tommy didn't budge, but as the cannula entered his trachea, he took a long deep breath, and I could feel him relaxing. His color immediately improved, and as he was wheeled out of the OR to where his mother waited, he was fast asleep

After I had been in practice about ten years, Mrs. Rossi, an expectant mother, came to visit me. The name struck a chord. Soon it dawned on me that this was the wife of the smoke shop owner who had taken my seven dollars when I was working for Coca-Cola many years ago. She seemed pleasant enough, and after our interview she decided that she would like me to be their pediatrician for the child she was expecting. I took care of that cute little baby and for all the other children they had in the ensuing years. However, on that first day after our meeting, I instructed my secretary that whenever we saw a child from that family for a professional reason, she was to add seven dollars to the bill.

All house calls were not created equal. Indeed, some were beyond my furthest imagination. One very hot summer evening, a house call came in from one of my younger, very attractive mothers at about 9:00 p.m. She told the answering service that her baby was crying with an ear ache. Upon arrival at the house I could hear music playing—belly dancing music—and I noticed that the lights in the house were dim.

Mrs. Manson greeted me at the door in a pink satin robe, gaping provocatively. The room behind her was dark except for the flickering of candles placed on a couple of tables in the room.

I stepped inside.

I heard the door lock behind me..

"Where's the baby?" I asked.

She smiled seductively and replied, "Upstairs, doc."

She led me upstairs to the master bedroom where the baby lay on an open queen sized bed, sleeping on the exposed satin sheets.

I checked the baby over and could find nothing wrong. I told her I thought the baby was well and perhaps had had a little gas, but was okay now.

"I didn't think so," she smiled. She rubbed her breast against me so I could smell the Chanel Number 5, and then, "Why not come downstairs with me and have a drink and fool around a little?" she asked provocatively.

I stood there looking at this twenty-plus gorgeous brunette with beautiful brown eyes and luscious lips just begging to make love, her hips moving slowly, and her mouth slightly open and moist, inviting, and eager.

I could feel manly things starting to happen to me.

"Thank you very much, but I have another house call to make," I lied. At the door, she embraced me in one last attempt before she unlocked the door and thanked me for coming. Phew!

On all future calls to her house—and there were a couple—I'd have the answering service call there thirty minutes from the time I left to make the call.

Al, my barber, had been born in Italy, and had become an American citizen by serving in the U.S. Marines. There is absolutely no prouder an American than one who becomes a citizen by serving in the Marines. When Al decided to get married, he went back to Italy. He found his bride, brought her home, and returned to his business. In a short while she was pregnant and had her first baby: a boy.

The first morning after the baby was born, I paid a visit to her and congratulated her on her fine boy. The young bride spoke very little English. With a little sign language and a lot of questions, I asked her if she would like him circumcised. This question was demonstrated with a vigorous chop down near the crotch. She was horrified and said, "No, doctor, donta cut!"

That night at visiting hours the horrified woman anxiously told her husband what had happened. He evidently told her that all Americans were circumcised, and his son was an American, and so, by God, the child would be circumcised.

The next morning when I went in to see her, she said, "You know, doctor, I beena tinkin abouta whatta you calla circumacision, and I'ma decide you canna do the job, but pleasa Doc, justa take a little offa da top and nuttin offa da sides."

I did my best to accommodate her wishes and to guarantee Al that he would be proud of his American son.

One bright and sunny fall day, only God knows why, but for some strange reason I had gotten to hospital about ten minutes earlier than usual. I went into the nursery and found two other pediatricians already there, too. They were discussing a fascinating case of a child whose father was in the Army Nike Missile unit stationed in our city.

The Army had taken over the old Town Farm for their headquarters, but some of them were married and others were placed in homes where there were extra rooms. (My parents had four of them staying in the two bedrooms and bath on the third floor). Other families with children were renting apartments all over the area.

One of these families had brought their nine-year-old girl to those two pediatricians with the story that she would get up every morning in fine spirits, have breakfast, get on the school bus, and go to school. Upon arriving at school she would within the hour of arrival, fall unconscious to the floor. She had been doing this since starting school when her parents were stationed in Europe. Both my friends were nonplussed, as had been the doctors in Europe.

That afternoon, I got a phone call from a woman asking to speak to me.

"Dr. Rackliffe? This is Mrs. Brotherton. I haven't met you yet, but my neighbor recommends you highly."

"What can I do for you, Mrs. Brotherton?"

"It's about my nine year-old daughter Linda. Ever since she started school in Europe, she has been having episodes of going unconscious after getting to school, and no one has been able to figure out what is going on. She had another one today."

"Is she awake now?"

"No sir. She hasn't moved since I bought her home from school. It's like this every time."

"All right. Take her to the Emergency Room at New Britain General and I will have her admitted."

"Yes sir. Thank you, doctor."

I called the admitting office at the hospital and had her admitted to my service, and then I called my favorite neurosurgeon, Jim Collias, and told him the story, including what I had overheard in the morning at the nursery, and asked him to take a look.

Jim got up there before I did, as he was through his office hours earlier, and was just finishing his exam when I arrived. The little girl was beginning to stir and make noises.

"Hi, Bob. I'm all done here, and I can't find anything wrong with her neurologically," said Jim.

I started my exam as Jim watched, and I could find nothing at all abnormal. In my mind I started down a lot of possibilities which ended up at dead ends, but suddenly, just like several times in the past when I was literally praying for an answer, I heard my voice say, "Who gave you the pills?"

Jim looked at me quizzically.

"My mommy told me not to tell anyone."

Thanks for that, Lord, I thought to myself. That thought would never have entered my mind.

I ordered a toxicology screen and the drug was Phenobarbital, which the mother gave to her just before she got on the school bus.

I then had two obligations: First to report this to the administration of the hospital. The other was to call the father and ask him to come up to the hospital tell him this most unlikely story.

When he arrived and had heard the story, he stared at me in disbelief, and then started to cry. Instinctively, I put my arm around his shoulder as he cried; sobbing against my body, he seemed unable to focus on what had transpired. He watched helplessly as the police came and arrested his wife, and listened while she denied everything, and then threatened to sue me and the hospital. As she was led away she became more agitated and incoherent. He watched her leave as he stayed by the bed of his little girl.

It was sad to see the father standing there watching the complete mental collapse of his wife. The thought that she might have killed their daughter was so awful to think about that I prayed she would be cured completely.

And a pparently she was. She was committed to the Brattleboro Hospital for the Insane, where her husband told me she was doing fine and they expected her to do well.

Upon return to practice in New Britain, I had every other weekend and every other night off, and four weeks a year for vacations. Lest you think it was all work and no play, let me assure you with four young boys ranging in age from four to twelve that was never the case. In the winters we skied, and in the summer we camped.

We used the vacation time to do something as a family. For summer use, I bought a Heilite camper, which was the size of a double bed. It was a double-hitched and single-wheel tent trailer, and when attached to the wagon it pulled easily at any speed. It opened up into two rooms twenty-one feet long; one room contained the double bed in the bed of the trailer, and had room for two cots, while the other room took two cots or three, if necessary. It had, under the bed of the camper, a pull-out kitchen, which consisted of an ice box, bread box, pantry area and a two burner Coleman stove. All the windows had nylon mesh screens with canvas pull-down sides, in the event of needing privacy or if it rained.

Every camping trip, we would leave with our four boys and usually a fifth (one of their friends). Jane and I had a pretty set routine that worked like a charm. We would arrive at a campground, and after having picked out the campsite, we would unhitch the camper and say, "Okay, guys. We're going for groceries and ice; have it all set up when we get back."

They would set to work, and they got so they were even putting up the tarpaulin that covered the table without any assistance from us. That tarp to cover the picnic table was fifteen feet square, and the boys would start with a pole centered on the picnic table while each of the kids would take a pole at a corner of the tarp and stake it into the ground, then they would stake the center poles on each side. This was the center of outdoor activity; meals, reading, cards, and board games. Two sides of this tarp had drop-down canvas sides which were tied, rolled up against the tarp, ready to be dropped in case of rain.

On our trips, we left with five or six boys, everything stowed in the camper and packed in our Studebaker station wagon. It had a Packard V-8 engine that was very powerful. We took that trailer on trips all over the northeast, to an island off the coast of Maine where we snorkeled for lobsters, and to a more organized camping area in Maine where we set up one time just off the beach. Next to us, on our left side, was a family from Massachusetts. They were bordering the private property to their left.

When we got there, Jane and I did our disappearing act, and when we got back the tent was all set, including the tarp. One evening there was a scream from the Massachusetts side. "Daddy! Daddy! Robbie fell through the cesspool on the private land." Quick as a flash, his dad was on his feet, took his pipe out of his mouth and shouted, "Keep your mouth shut, Robbie!"

Good advice.

Well-when that kid came out and came into view, I was so glad he wasn't mine!

One year we camped on Prince Edward Island. The water was as warm as Florida, courtesy of the Gulf Stream, and the soil was red from the iron content. By then we had become a convoy with two other families from New Britain camping with us. One of the other families had four boys and one girl. The other family had two more boys. that totaled ten boys and one girl. The waterfront at that camp was a nice red sandy beach and, anchored off shore, a raft. One day the raft broke loose from its mooring and had to be shoved out to be reattached, I took a picture of ten boys on the raft and one girl in the water, pushing.

As I watched this amusing spectacle, I wondered at what age the latent feminism would come forth. Somewhere along the path of life, that schema gets properly arranged, emphatically and unequivocally.

The Hagedorns were the family with the five kids, and they were patients of mine. coincidentally, my sons had been patients of Dr. Hagedorn, an orthopedic surgeon of great renown in New Britain. He took care of Jimmy's and Dannie's broken legs (two at the same time from ski mishaps). Max knew absolutely nothing about camping, but he loved his children so much that when his wife suggested that they try camping with us, he agreed. They arrived a day or two after us, and he set up his tent with the help of his four boys, while his wife Marie and their daughter Mary looked on. They pitched their tent on a slight slope but it seemed okay when it was finally up.

That night it started to rain, and in the morning Max asked me to look over their tent situation. As I approached the tent I could hear a gurgling sound. When I got there, I could see why. There was a two-inch wide stream of water in a slight trench rumbling down towards and under the middle of the tent, and exiting on the lower side. Standing in the doorway you could see the stream running under the tent floor—right through the middle of the tent.

Oh how I laughed! Max looked at me, smiled and shrugged.

"No problem, Max. We just have to make a trench to divert the stream. Do you have a shovel?"

Of course he didn't. What would you need a shovel for?

"Jim, go back to our camp and get our trenching tool and you and the other guys here fix it, okay?"

"Sure, Dad."

"Max, why don't you and Marie come down to our camp and have a cup of coffee while the boys are fixing this?"

"Sounds good to me!" laughed Marie.

We wandered down to our camp, laughing about the scene on the tent floor, and when we told Jane what was going on, she burst out laughing with the rest of us. The coffee was hot and delicious!

Now I understood the true meaning of "tenderfoot."

A few days later, we were scheduled to part company. We were heading for Nova Scotia and the Cabot trail, and the other two families were heading home. The boys packed their clothes and stowed their bags in the trailer under the double bed. Then they let down the tent, folding the two sections on top of the double bed. Last to go on was the folded picnic tarp, its poles, and the spare tire for the trailer wheel. Then the cover was snapped all around the periphery of the trailer, making all secure and set to go.

We said our good byes to the Hagedorns and the other couple, Bob and Grace Ingerson and their two sons, started that lovely V8 engine, and pulled away on a Sunday morning. I marveled at the effortless power in that great little wagon.

Our plan was to drive east to the ferry that regularly plied its way between Prince Edward Island and Nova Scotia. From there we would be landing on the western side of Nova Scotia. Our campground was in the provincial park on Cape Breton, which was the northeast corner Nova Scotia. It would take a few hours to get from the landing in Nova Scotia to Cape Breton.

We figured to have breakfast in Nova Scotia, pulling over at some picnic site and making breakfast. That plan faded from view in the wake of the departing ferry, which we had missed by a matter of minutes. It would be two hours before it returned.

We were first in line for the next ferry on a beautiful, warm, sunny Sunday, with water on three sides of us, and a rapidly increasing line of cars coming to a halt behind us to await the next ferry.

Time for breakfast! Dan and Jim pulled out the kitchen from the side of the trailer, lowered the front legs so that it was stable and started the burners on the stove. Peter put the toaster on one burner and four slices of bread at a time on a frame over the burner. They toasted quickly over the open flame, and he was busy turning them to toast the other side. In no time at all, enough toast was done and Jim put the bacon in the frying pan while the percolator went on the other burner. Jane did the eggs after the bacon, and they were soon ready. It smelled so good on that pier that everyone's tongue was hanging out. The food was delicious out there in the warm sunshine, and there were many envious people standing around smelling that super breakfast. We did make an extra pot of coffee for some adults, but we were also in need of a grocery stop when we got over to Cape Breton.

I have never, ever had a more scrumptious breakfast. Both Jane and I felt very bad that we didn't have enough food or even toast to share with the people there; aside from the coffee, we were down to practically only what we had saved for breakfast, and we planned to restock a lot before heading onto the cape, where no supplies would be available.

We had plenty of time to clean up and stow everything away as we watched, over a second cup of coffee, the ferry coming back for the next load. When the ferry docked and prepared to load us, the tide was right so that the dock and the ferry was level and we just drove on. *Piece of cake!* I thought.

The trip over to Cape Breton took about two hours. As we approached the unloading pier there, I could see that we had a problem. The dock and the ferry were not at the same level, so twelve-inch-wide planks were lowered onto the ferry and I was told to drive up the planks, a change in height of about four feet. "We'll take care of baby!" shouted one of the deck hands, and as I drove up the ramp, a couple of them lifted the rear end of the trailer and the center mounted fifteen-inch wheel, for which there was no plank, and walked our trailer off the boat, plopping our little fifth wheel ("the baby") on dry land. Just like that.

At the first town we found a grocery store, and I was delighted to see he had everything we needed to restock, including ice. The gray-haired kindly old man asked, "Where are you headed?"

"We're on our way to the provincial park on Cape Breton, sir," I replied.

"Suppose you're planning to drive around the Cabot Trail."

"Yes sir, we are. Do you have any suggestions?"

"Yes I do. Drive around the trail counter-clockwise. That way you are hanging right over the cliffs. Much better view going that way."

"Thanks for the advice, sir. How long is it from here to the provincial park?"

"Couple of hours will put you right at the entrance. You and your young family have a good time up there," he said.

"Thank you, sir." I paid him for the groceries and ice, and we started back on our way.

In just about two hours, we were heading north towards Cape Breton, when we saw signs announcing the Provincial Park on either side of the road. The two-lane road was excellent, and the terrain was untouched with sharp rock outcroppings surrounded by towering pines. The air smelled of balsam and salt sea. Below us and on the right side of the car it was a sheer drop to the ocean, but as we proceeded, the land on the right kept increasing in distance until it too was pine covered, and jagged gray rock was evident everywhere, with the ocean in the distance.

As we turned a corner on our way, we gazed in awe at a vast expanse of beautiful green lawn, mowed to perfection, and dotted with trellises which were ablaze with different colored roses; fish pools with statuary framed a black entranceway to an English Tudor building of about forty rooms.

The driveway curved in a graceful circle in front of the entrance. There was a large black limousine parked in front of the imposing main entrance, and in a parking lot to one side were many expensive cars.

It was beautiful to see the white stucco building with frames of dark oak showing and a light brown roof overhanging it. I counted four chimneys, each of which had four stacks rising from the brick.

A very dignified dark green sign hanging from a white post and support announced quietly in gold gilt that this was the "Celtic Lodge."

It reeked of money.

Finally we came to the campground, which was a huge field of grass and wildflowers carved out of a forest of pines. In the center there was a manager's office and toilet and shower buildings for both sexes. Stretching out from these buildings on both sides were tents, tent trailers like ours, and several deluxe trailers that were like miniature homes. Some even had air conditioning. There was also a row for RVs.

We found our assigned lot, and everyone pitched in to erect the tarp over the picnic table, level the camper, and fetch water so that in no time, we were all set. We checked out the camp store where the selection was sparse and expensive.

The next morning there were a man and a child standing quietly at the edge of our space. "Doc?" he asked when I came out of the tent, "Could you look at my son? He's complaining of an earache."

"Sure I can, but how did you know that I was a doctor?"

"One of the campers here was on the ferry with you and saw your MD license plate," he replied. (These had always been an advantage when making house calls, as the police looked the other way if parking rules were being violated.)

"Well, let's have a look." I checked the lad's ears and he had an acute infection in one of them. It must have been a long night for the poor little guy.

I gave him some medicine for it. (I always carried medicines and suture material with us. I even had a bottle of Morphine; (why I had it I don't know; I usually did not carry anything stronger than codeine.)

They had a golf course there in the Provincial Park, and we had heard that it was quite different, so one of the first days we were there we went to play nine holes, taking the boys along with us. It was different all right. I have never seen anything like it in all my golfing experience. Standing on the first tee the only thing you could see was a very dense forest and one golf hole. There was the fragrant smell of balsam everywhere, and along the sides of the hole, wildflowers were in abundance.

The woods were alive with sounds; birds singing as if in a contest, and we heard a bone-chilling scream of a bobcat (I think!?) up in the height of one of the taller trees. When we arrived at the green, the next tee was visible, but nothing else except more woods. When we had finished, we had played nine holes without ever seeing any other hole except the one we were on, and it had been a nature walk for all of us. The golf turned out to be incidental.

Next day, one of my boys had an infection on one toe that was looking pretty ugly so I went over to the camp store for some Bacitracin ointment.

"We don't have anything like that here but you can get it in a town called Neil's Harbor, where there is a hospital and doctor thirty-five miles north of here. The doc up there is a young guy, and his name is Dr. Lowell."

So after seeing three sick kids standing outside my tent, I put in a call for Dr. Lowell. He answered the phone himself. "Neil's Harbor Hospital, Dr. Lowell speaking."

"Dr. Lowell, this is Dr. Rackliffe calling. I am staying at the Provincial Campground here, and I was wondering if you had any Bacitracin ointment available?

"Yes, I do, Doctor, and if you come up here, I will be glad to make it available to you. What kind of a doctor are you?"

"A pediatrician," I replied.

"Great! I will be glad to help you out, and if you will, I would like you to see four kids I have in the hospital here. They all have gastroenteritis, and I am a little shaky on IV fluid management in kids."

"I'll be happy to see them with you," I said. "We'll be leaving here within ten minutes or so. I would imagine we should be there within the hour."

We all piled in the car and drove thirty-five miles up the Cabot Trail to Neil's Harbor Hospital, which was right on the only street going through the town.

Dr. Lowell greeted me at the door of the small two-story hospital made of stone. Outside the back of the hospital, one could see the ocean hitting the rocks of the shore several hundred feet below us.

The little hospital had two wings off the main central entrance. The odor of ether was very noticeable, mixed with another familiar scent: Lysol. Dr. Lowell showed me the operating/delivery room and an empty patient's room on the left side, and then we headed for the right side of the hospital, which had a couple of patient's rooms.

Lastly, we came to a pediatric ward with beds and curtains on tracks to give them privacy when needed. There were four children ranging from age two to five years in four of the eight beds provided. They were all hooked up to IVs and looked pretty sick.

"They have all been here for three days. None of them is from the same family, and they all are from town here. No one has had a fever greater than 101, but they are pretty worn out from the diarrhea, and I just don't know if I'm giving them the right stuff. Stool cultures came back this morning and they are negative."

"Well let's have a look at them," I said and we started down the line with me examining all of them from top to toe. Aside from dehydration in varying degrees amongst the four of them, I could find no other pathology.

"I think what you need is a method of calculating fluid requirements for kids according to their size. Let me give you some numbers and solution mixtures so that you will feel more comfortable handling these little guys when they come in."

After about a half hour, I had prepared a treatment regimen complete with fluids to use, how much, and when to add oral fluids for him to use. I also gave him a formula so that he could make an oral electrolyte replacement solution out of what he would always be able to obtain, even there in the boondocks.

As we finished up and I was preparing to leave, I asked him for the tube of Bacitracin.

He handed me a tube and then said, "That'll be $2.75."

I couldn't believe that after spending two hours or so helping him out of a hole and smoothing his path for the future, he would charge me for the ointment. But there he stood, waiting for me to pay him.

So he got his $2.75 from one unhappy colleague. Where I came from physicians didn't charge physicians.

When I came down the steps of the hospital, the boys all cheered and Jimmy said, "Finally!" This prompted Stevie to echo, "Yeah, Dad, finally."

Jane said, "We have walked all over this village looking for something to do, and they have been getting pretty restless. Thank goodness we had the Frisbee with us. Even some of the local kids joined in when the boys were playing with that, until one of them threw it up there." She pointed to the roof of the hospital, and there in the rain gutter was a flash of yellow plastic.

There was no place to get a bite for lunch, so we headed back to the camp hungry and frustrated. But at least we had the Bacitracin for Peter's toe.

As we arrived at the campground, I drove down to our site, and after parking the car, noticed the shiny black limousine at the camp office CELTIC LODGE" was emblazoned on the driver's door in gold letters.

Jane had the coffee going, and Jim was buttering the bread for sandwiches. Stevie was setting the table, and Danny had gone for water, and I was working on Peter's infected foot. I happened to look up to see the manager of the campground and a man in a chauffeur's uniform approaching me.

The camp manager came directly to me and said, "Doctor, there is a very sick man over at the lodge, and they called the doctor up at Neil's Harbor. He said to ask you to look at him and then call him."

Rats! I got my bag, got in the limo, and was driven into this super-upper-crust establishment in my shorts and golf shirt, and was shown into the gentleman's room. He looked terrible! He was obviously in great pain.

The history was that he had gotten a belly ache and fever four days prior, and the pain had eventually gone down to the right lower quadrant of his abdomen. When I felt his abdomen, it was as I expected: board-like and very painful to the touch. I listened to the distended abdomen, and it was silent. He had peritonitis from a ruptured appendix. I called our hero in Neil's Harbor and told him the facts and that he needed to go to a hospital yesterday or sooner. He asked me if I had anything for pain, and I admitted that I had a bottle of morphine in my possession, but I was not a licensed Canadian physician and would not use it unless he ordered it.

"Use it- give him quarter grain IM, and I will have a helicopter pick him up and get him to Halifax right away." So I gave him a quarter grain of morphine and within an hour he was on his way.

Thank God I had that morphine!

The next morning there were fourteen people waiting in line by my picnic tarp when we got up. This was ridiculous! I was the only doctor within thirty-five miles in a tourist summer hot spot. I did what I could for them. It was mostly minor stuff, but the problem was the lack of a pharmacy for the simplest of medications.

It was frustrating to see five kids with ear infections and not be able to give them a prescription to run down to a local pharmacy, rather than going all the way to Neil's Harbor for a prescription of Amoxicillin (which I wasn't sure they would get from Dr. Lowell).

There were four or five kids with pretty heavy cases of poison ivy that I recommended they use a salt solution in compresses and expose to the air between compresses. Some of the campers had Calamine lotion with them, which I suggested they share with each other. I did not see one case of swimmer's ear, simply because they were swimming in salt water, and swimmer's ear is not a saltwater ailment. It is a disease coming from bacterially contaminated pool or lake water, frequently held in the victim's ear by a large accumulation of ear wax for a long enough time to create the condition.

Of the remaining kids, one had a laceration that needed suturing, and because only twelve hours had elapsed since it had happened, I used some of my suture material and put in four stitches, without anesthesia, in the leg of a very brave little six-year-old boy, who didn't so much as whimper. When I was through suturing, I sewed the needle and thread that was left on his shirt for all to see, which pleased him greatly. That left a couple of kids with diarrhea, who weren't so bad that they needed IVs, so I gave their parents my magic oral electrolyte formula to make for them.

So about eleven o'clock that day, we were finally free to do something as a family. Up until that time the boys and Jane had been waiting for me to be free. Jane and I talked the situation over. It was obvious that the whole time there would be consumed by the needs of the many tourists who were nearby and needed medical help, which I was unable to do due to lack of supplies, so we decided to cut our stay short there, making the trip home more leisurely.

We talked it over with the boys to see how they felt about it and asked them what they wanted to do.

In a chorus, "Yeah, Dad! Let's pack up and leave. Mom's been looking in the camping book, and there is a place called Moose Horn Wildlife refuge in Maine that looks cool!"

"Okay, let's do it!" I said, after a nod from Jane. "Break camp!" It was organized chaos. All clothes were packed in the six carry-ons and put in the trailer under the bed and next to the kitchen, which was already stowed. Peter and Steve started pulling stakes and folding the tent down on our bed, followed rapidly by the second section that made up the other room.

Then the whole family started pulling stakes and grabbing tent poles as we took down the tarp, folded it, and laid it atop the folded tent on top of the tent poles. Last thing on was the spare trailer tire, which disappeared under the trailer cover as it was snapped all around to its fasteners.

By the time we finished we had quite an audience of campers, and we did the whole job in less than a half hour.

As we all piled into the car, there was many a "Good bye" and "Thanks, Doc!" as we slowly pulled away waving to the many new friends we had made.

The sign announcing the entrance to the Moose Horn Wild Life Refuge was as big as a billboard and depicted a very large moose with a huge rack coming at us. It was wild all right. There was no building anywhere, and the road was dirt and wound through the trees and meadows. Jane picked out the campsite (as she always did), and as we started to set up, I realized that the five-gallon water container was almost empty.

"Come on Pete, let's you and I find some water."

"Okay, Pop," replied Peter, and the two of us set out to find a water pipe like several we had seen jutting out of the ground randomly as we drove in. We started down a dirt road opposite our campsite expecting to come upon a water faucet somewhere, in Maine parlance, "down the road a piece."

Well that "piece" turned out to be at least a quarter mile away.

The steel container was square with many sharp edges, and the handle was the size of a suitcase handle welded to the center of the square top. It held five gallons when full; that's forty pounds plus the weight of the container.

It wasn't heavy at all as we proceeded to look for a faucet, but when we filled it up and started back down the road, we probably hadn't gone more than a hundred yards when that handle was hurting like hell. I switched to the other hand. Then Peter tried and we got a little further, but it was cruel work.

"Dad, why don't we find a stick and put it through the handle and then we can both carry it."

"Great idea, Peter."

We started looking for a stick less than an inch in diameter because there was only an inch clearance between the handle and the tank.

Peter found one that looked pretty good and it fit under the handle, so we both took hold and lifted.

Snap! It broke in half, and the tank crashed to the ground landing on one corner which bent but did not leak, thank God. Next, Peter found three smaller but stronger branches that were not deadwood, which we threaded through the handle space and carefully tested. Nothing broke, although they bent a little.

We slowly made our way back to camp without the sticks breaking, and having to pause to ease the discomfort on our hands a couple of times, but we got there.

We started to tell the others about our difficult trip and the pain and effort involved, and Danny broke into a big smile and started to laugh.

"What the hell is so funny?" I fumed.

"Dad, let me show you something," he said as he continued to laugh heartily. He walked towards a little shrub about forty to fifty feet from the campsite, pulled the shrub aside, and pointed. A water faucet leered at us.

I looked at Peter, and he looked at me as I spoke for both of us. "Shit!"

Peter smiled.

Next day we left Moose Horn after finding the water there equally as cold as that on Cape Breton, and the beach more rocks than sand. The only wildlife we saw was the moose on the billboard at the entrance.

We traversed the length of Maine, and then pulled in to a campground built off the Maine highway by the state as a convenience to travelers. We were set up in a matter of minutes, not bothering with the tarp because it was a lovely night, and no rain was expected. After breakfast in the morning, we repacked and took off for home arriving in the mid-afternoon.

First thing on the menu was to go get the dogs out of the keeper's kennels, after which we were once again a complete family with lots of happy memories.

Winter weekends were ski weekends whenever I was not on call. To really capitalize on good skiing, we bought an old house in Bondville, Vermont, that came furnished. The house, which was known locally as the Landerman Place, was right on route 30 and at the base of Stratton Mountain.

Nearby was a new development of ski chalets where our friends the Brays, Waskowitzes, and the Fletchers, and a couple of other New Britain families had places, so weekends were always pleasant, skiing with friends and picnicking on the mountain if it were not too cold.

One of the happiest moments of my life occurred one Easter Sunday morning when I was skiing along a ridge at the top of Mt. Snow, with three of my sons behind me. It was warm and sunny, and I felt a poke in my rear end from a ski pole. I stopped and turned to see my three sons lined out behind me, like little ducks, all smiling. Jimmy, in the lead said, "Gee, Dad, this is fun!" That's a memory I will always cherish.

One year early on in our skiing history, there was forecast for snow on a Wednesday. I had Wednesdays off, so I declared the First Annual Rackliffe Hooky Day for the next day.

We drove up to Vermont Tuesday night and were ready for skiing by eight in the morning. Hooky days became an annual event. One year the boys claimed another hooky day because on the day I had selected, schools were closed due to snow.

In another year, we had two broken legs at the same time, both gotten on hooky days. It was kind of funny seeing the tutors greeting each other as they came and went.

The attitude of the teachers was interesting. One older teacher encouraged us to have these special days as family, while the younger one was not happy about the kids playing hooky and even less happy that it was done with the parent's permission.

Jane and I had no regrets or feelings of guilt. We both thought the older teacher was great. This was good for the family, and we knew it.

PART 9:

KLINGBERG CHILDREN'S HOME

O ne of the plans I had in my head when I finally opened an office to practice pediatrics was to offer my services—free—to the Klingberg Children's home. I wanted to do that because it meant that I would be the third generation of my family to be of help to them. Klingberg was a fascinating place and its history even more so.

In 1915, a minister from a Swedish church was walking in the down town area of New Britain when he was hailed by a big, burly policeman who had hold of a small boy in each hand."Pastor, could you take care of these little tykes? They've got no home." So John Klingberg brought them home, and when his wife objected, asking where the money to feed them would come, Pastor Klingberg reassured her: "God will provide."

He had come from poverty in Sweden and had been in New Britain less than five years when the two little boys were brought to him. He considered their being brought to him as a commission from God.

He was a big raw boned man whose eyeglasses were always perched halfway down his large, rather prominent nose. He had a hearty laugh and always wore a smile on his face. He was as easy to love as he was loving. Everyone in town knew him and also knew what he was doing: He was trusting God to meet their needs. He never asked anyone for money or food or clothes, but prayed, confident that God would see his needs and provide.

After making the commitment to accept those two little boys, he and his wife opened their home to other children, and in a short time the Klingbergs were caring for twenty-seven needy ones in their home on Garden Street.

One Sunday when the family and the children sat down to lunch there was no food in the house. Pastor Klingberg started saying grace for what they were about to receive. In the middle of his prayer there was a knock on the front door. On the porch next to the door were four baskets of food from a bartender's picnic that had been rained out.

As people became aware of what was going on, they tried to help this unique man who thanked God for everything and never doubted there would be enough.

The actions of the Swedish pastor intrigued one of the wealthy men in town to the point that he called Pastor Klingberg. "Reverend Klingberg? This is Howard Platt, and I have been hearing so many tales about you and what you are doing, that I would like to meet you."

"Certainly Mr. Platt, I would be delighted to meet with you at your convenience. When would be a time that would suit you?"

"How about tomorrow at my house?" said Mr. Platt.

"That would be fine. One o'clock all right with you?"

So the two men sat down on the porch of Mr. Platt's house and discussed what Pastor Klingberg was doing and what his dreams and hopes were for the future.

Pastor Klingberg explained how he had started with the two little boys found abandoned and what happened then. "I suddenly felt as though a hand had been put on my shoulder and a voice said to me: 'Take these children and I will send you more and you will provide for them.' I felt directed by God." The big man paused, then smiled and said, "Now we are up to twenty-seven"

"Tell me, Reverend, how do you think you are going to manage this? It's obviously growing by leaps and bounds. What are you going to do next? You need more room. What you need is land to build an orphanage. Is that the way you are thinking?"

John Klingberg sat quietly rocking in his chair. "That would be a wonderful solution, Mr. Platt. God gave me those children to care for, and he has sent me twenty-five more in the past two years. It is his will that my wife and I care for them. Anything we need has come to us by just praying and believing that God will provide. If it is his will for us to build an orphanage, it will happen."

As Pastor Klingberg got up to leave, Mr. Platt shook his hand and said: "Reverend Klingberg, you are an inspiration, and I am going to try and help you in every way I can. I thank you for your time, and I assure you, you will hear from me again."

"Thank you for seeing me, sir, and God be with you," replied pastor Klingberg.

Unbeknownst to Klingberg, Mr. Platt then started looking for available land for the orphanage. He noticed there was a farm on the top of one of the city's hills known as Rackliffe Heights in the southern end the city. It was part of my grandfather's farm. My dad used to go up there every day and "slop" the pigs when he was a boy. (That had to be one hell of a job carrying food up that steep hill every day.)

Mr. Platt approached my grandfather about the land and told him why he was looking for land. He asked, "Would you be interested in selling it, Frank?"

"Well, since my brothers and I started the hardware business, I haven't been using that hill except for the hogs, and if you say Reverend Klingberg is an honest man and is looking to build a children's home, I reckon he can have the land for what I owe in back taxes on it, which is somewhere around $2,200."

"That's mighty generous of you, Frank" said Mr. Platt.

I think my grandfather was impressed with Pastor Klingberg's mission and Howard Platt's request. The fact that Howard's brother, Fred, had financed Rackliffe Bros. Co. Inc. probably was a factor, too.

So Pastor Klingberg started planning his children's home and a farm on Rackliffe Heights. Although it is one of the highest hills in the city, the terrain was rounded and contained a lot of good farmland as well as being level on the top so building was not a challenge. The hill over looked the city and was an ideal spot for a children's home, being less than a mile from the elementary school and less than a mile from the hospital in town.

On the west side the property overlooked Doerr's Pond from which the Doerr family cut ice every winter. The ice was stored in an ice house standing alongside the pond on Shuttle Meadow Avenue, right across the street from the Vance elementary school.

Howard Platt, the man who made all of these plans come to fruition after talking with Pastor Klingberg and my grandfather, was considered by his family as the "black sheep" because he played golf on Sunday, did not attend church, and made his living speculating in real estate.

He was extremely successful in business, and when he died he left his substantial fortune entirely to the Klingberg Children's Home.

For my family's part, when my father took over the business, any item needed by the home was supplied either free or, with big purchases like tractors, at our cost.

From the beginning of his orphanage, Pastor Klingberg was opposed to separating siblings, in the event that there was no parent or relative to take care of them. He wanted them all or none. In that way, they still had a sense of family within the family at the home.

Work was started immediately to build the orphanage on the top of the hill, and it sat there welcoming the children to a single story building that had a porch covering most of the front of the building, complete with rocking chairs. The interior of the building had offices lining the front wall with entrances from a building-long hallway. On the opposite wall of the hallway were a boys' ward and bathrooms on one end, next to that was the dining hall, then the assembly hall, and finally the girls' ward and bathrooms. The possessions of each child were kept in bureaus at the head of each bed.

There was no privacy. A proctor's room was situated in each dormitory for supervision and provided an adult for emergencies.

In just a few years there was a working farm going on the hill. There was a barn, milk cows, chickens, beef cattle, as well as hogs and a huge vegetable garden. All of the children were involved in helping to run it. Some of the boys came from places in the States where they had already milked cows, so they were put on that duty and were required to teach the other boys who milked the cows twice a day. The smaller boys were responsible for feeding them and slopping their stalls and also were responsible for the care of the hogs, as well as the two draft horses they used to plow the garden. Pastor Klingberg hired a farmer to oversee the farm and live on the property.

Girls were responsible for caring for the chickens and collecting the eggs.

Everyone—including the very smallest (two- and three-year-olds) were involved in the vegetable garden. The garden was huge and had every edible vegetable or fruit growing in it, in well weeded, wonderful soil. The children were especially diligent around the cantaloupe and watermelon patches, as well as the strawberry patch. I suspect the strawberry patch didn't yield as much as anticipated due to tasty plump berries picked by hungry hands.

As the fame of the orphanage grew in 1943, there was an article in *Reader's Digest* called, "The House that Prayer Built." Since this magazine was printed in twenty-plus languages and distributed world wide, the article prompted a deluge of two things: children and gifts. One gift was of sixty acres of land in Tucson, Arizona. This was willed to the home, to be conveyed when the owner died, and in the 1940s was described as arid land and sagebrush.

In 1946, Dr. John Klingberg died, leaving the orphanage leaderless. Of his three sons, one, Rev. Haddon Klingberg, along with his wife Myrtle, gave up a church ministry in the Midwest and came home to run the Children's Home. He did not enjoy the children to the extent his father had, but he accepted the charge. He continued the rule of asking only God for sustenance.

In a way the difference between the two men was as if God had planned it. The father John loved the children and gave them security, love, and a happy growing experience, for he had a great sense of humor and shared it with his children. Trusting in God, he started the home, but he was not a business man in any sense of the word.

His son Haddon, while religious and a good man, did not have the enthusiastic love for children that was John's hallmark. However, he was a businessman and a builder. One of his first moves was to appoint a volunteer board of directors, which included a stock broker named Ernest Brainard who willingly managed the stocks and income of the home. Because people all over the world had heard the story of the "house that prayer built," there was a steady flow of donations of money, securities, and land from everywhere.

Even in his nineties, Mr. Brainard, this wonderful man, continued to manage the home's portfolio. His interest in the home was unlimited. In summer he would go picking blueberries and after laboring all afternoon in the field would bring up a huge bucket of them for the kids. He was also an expert clock smith, and kept all the clocks running for the home and for his friends.

Once I asked him how to make money in the market. He smiled angelically and said, "Sell when everyone is buying and buy when everyone is selling."

As the fame of the Klingberg orphanage became increasingly known, especially the continued reliance on God as their sole source of sustenance and care, the home was held in ever greater respect. There was great approval of the fact that the sibling orphans would remain together. More and more children were being flown there from all over the United States. They came from Baptist churches mostly, sibling orphans from catastrophic family problems, such as death of a parent, parents being sent to prison, insanity of one parent, desertion. All sorts of sad stories came with the children. A few of the children were from the surrounding cities and towns, but most came from other states through the Baptist Church network.

When I returned to my hometown, it was perfectly natural, therefore, to want to follow my grandfather's gift of land to this Klingberg orphanage, my father's gift of any and all of their hardware needs, with my gift of service. Growing up, I had had many of the children from there as friends and schoolmates of mine. I loved the idea of being the physician for and loving those one hundred forty-seven children who had no parents and were so alone. I knew that my grandfather would have approved completely, and I just knew it was right for me—God given, I'd say. I called Haddon and made an appointment to meet with him.

We met at the home.

"What can I do for you, doctor?" he asked.

"Well, for one, you can call me Bob, but since my family has been involved with this home for two generations, I would like to offer my services for the care of the children free of charge."

"Thank you for that offer, Bob, and I am delighted to accept it. At the present time we are being taken care of by Dr. Bernstein, and he has been very generous with his time and attention, so I think that it might be proper for you to call him and explain your interest to him, and after you have done that, let me know and I will send him a letter of thanks. By the way, please call me Haddon."

"That's great. I will be here every Thursday morning to do physical exams on the kids—all of them so we will have a record of each child on file here in the infirmary."

"Why don't you join us for breakfast on Thursdays then?" Haddon asked.

Later that day I called Dwight Bernstein and explained the family connection and asked him if he would mind letting me take over their care.

"No, not at all. I've certainly got enough to do, and I would be happy for you to take over. It will help me slow down a little."

"Thanks for understanding, Dwight. I really am looking forward to it."

So it was agreed. Breakfast with the children was a very happy experience for me, and allowed me to get closer to them, and incidentally, reduce the fear of doctors that some of them had.

When Haddon accepted my offer, I had an immediate increase in number of patients in my practice of one hundred forty-seven new ones. Every Thursday morning I would go up and have breakfast with them.

Jane and I liked the idea that should anything happen to both parents, the children would be kept together, so we had our wills changed so that if anything happened to us simultaneously, our boys would have been taken care of together at the home.

Thanks to the management of the incoming funds by Ernie Brainard, there a new eight bed infirmary; four for boys, and four for girls, with the nurse's room in between. There was also an empty room in the infirmary, I noticed. At the end of the infirmary was a new two-story dormitory specifically built for taking care of two- to five-yearold children. Each bathtub was raised and had a kneeling pad around it. This section was staffed with very mother-like ladies and was a great improvement for the little ones. They all had bedrooms they shared with one other child.

The full time nurse who lived there was great. I gave her my home phone number, and also instructed the answering service to put their calls through to me, even if I were not on call. It turned out that I was up at the home about four to seven times per week.

Every Thursday at breakfast, I would sit at a different table and eat with the kids and chat and laugh with them, learn their names, and love them. When they came down to my office in the new infirmary for their physicals, I made sure they smiled and laughed, even if I had to tickle them, which was something I loved to do anyway. The nurse who was always there during my visits used to reassure them so that the whole experience was a happy one. Nobody ever left the exam frightened or crying, even if there were occasional immunizations given.

The first thing that struck me was the deplorable condition of the children's teeth. I asked a wonderful pediatric dentist if he would be willing to help out. (As there was an empty room in the infirmary, I was thinking of a dental office there.) Dr. Bill Morrissey was a super friendly, giving man who agreed to help with the dental needs of the children. One Thursday he, Haddon, and I walked through the infirmary to the empty room and talked about having the dental office there.

"How much would it cost?" asked Haddon.

Bill thought about it a bit and then said, "About $5,000." Bills eyes twinkled at the thought of putting in a pediatric dentist chair here, a sink over here. He was ready to go, and it showed with a big Irish grin on his face.

Haddon said: "I'll pray about it." That was a really noncommittal answer, and I was disappointed by his apparent lack of enthusiasm.

In the Monday mail was a check for $5,000. The dental clinic was built, under supervision from Bill, and he was happily in action within two months.

It was such a pleasure to examine the mouths of kids who had been to Bill before I got them. He did beautiful work.

After a few years, I was named to the board of trustees and served on that for twenty-seven years.

A piece of land of about ten acres was given to the Klingberg Home. Not having any need for it, they sold it for $40,000. The man who bought it sold just the topsoil off of it for $40,000, and one small piece of land at the edge of the property for $25,000. Two other much larger pieces went for $75,000 each. I remember when that happened thinking, *Why didn't we do those ourselves?*

One family of children was shipped in from Minnesota: one girl and two boys. Their mother died in childbirth and the father was in jail.

Every summer, a lot of families, sometimes distantly related, but often not, would take a child from the home on vacation with them. Clearly, the new family of four was not going to have any calls or invites from relatives, and since Jane and I had always wanted a girl, we decided to invite one of the new family's girls to go with us on our family summer vacation. We thought it would be a good experience for the boys, too.

Her name was Muriel, and we enjoyed her very much. She had been through so much and was so vulnerable, and had never felt an arm around her shoulders or a hug or kiss. We wanted her to feel those things, to feel like family, and to let her know that she was loved by us.

We knew we had succeeded when she asked Jane if she could call her "Mom."

She always called me "Doc." Being from the home and having two brothers, Muriel was used to boys, but she was a real novelty and a source of great curiosity to our four boys. The first vacation we went to Cape Cod. To my surprise Muriel was homesick for the home. I was amazed. How can you be homesick for an institution? She was, but after a few days of having fun in the waves and getting used to the four boys, the homesickness was a thing of the past, and she became family. The boys loved her and she went on vacations with us from that year on.

One year, we went to a lodge on Little Deer Isle in Maine, and when I made the reservation, I told them that we were bringing a girl from the Children's Home with us. The owner was Dr. Waldron who was the professor of botany at the University of Maine. He was fascinating to listen to, and we all spent two to three hours many times in our two weeks there in a meadow listening to him lecture and demonstrate what was right there at our feet that we didn't even see, much less know. This kindly scholar kept us looking at what appeared to be an ordinary hump of grass in a bog, pointing out the entire ecosystem that survived because of it.

He took us out to sail in the bay on his thirty-foot sailboat and had all the kids manning cleats, lines and sails, making sailors of them all.

When time came to go, I asked for my bill and it did not include Muriel. I pointed this out to the kind man, and he said: "You brought her here for me to touch and I thank you for the opportunity."

I felt the presence of God in this man.

The Children's Home took a lot of my time. There was scarcely a week that I was not up there more than just Thursday. There was always someone with a strep throat or croup, cough, rashes, even lacerations—if not too serious. There were a few children who broke their arms over time, and my friend, Dr. Bill Waskowitz, an orthopedic surgeon, graciously attended them.

Meanwhile, back at the office most days were pretty routine. but one afternoon in September, one of my moms named Meredith came in with her daughter Emily and announced, "I'm going to die."

"What are you talking about?" I asked. I put my arm around her shoulders and could feel the tension slowly soften as we talked.

She was a lovely, well educated woman, and I could see she was on the edge and resigned to her coming death, while her eyes had the look of a startled deer desperately looking for a way out.

"I have an inoperable aneurysm in my brain that's going to rupture some day, and I will be dead."

"Who says so?" I asked in disbelief.

"Both the neurosurgeons at Hartford and Boston say so. No one will operate on me, because they say the aneurysm is in a dangerous place, and almost inaccessible without damaging my brain irreparably."

Wow! The whole story shook me and yet it sounded familiar. Then I remembered that Bud Riley, farher of two boys that were patients of mine, had had an identical problem and had it fixed. I called him and asked about his surgery, and how he managed to get it fixed. It was an identical story to hers; refusal to operate both in Hartford and Boston, for fear that the operation would either kill him or leave him in a vegetative state.

Somehow he had heard of a neurosurgeon in Toronto, and had been successfully operated on there. I called Meredith, who was awaiting death, and told her about the neurosurgeon at Toronto General Hospital and suggested she call Dr. Jim Collias at Hartford Hospital and ask him to make the arrangements.

About two weeks later I was in one of the examining rooms, and my secretary called in to interrupt me, as there was a phone call for me. It was Meredith.

"Do you know where I am?" she asked.

"No. Where are you?"

"I'm at Toronto General." She purred, then, "Do you know what else?"

"No. What else?"

"I'm all fixed."

"Really! That's wonderful! Are you totally okay?"

"Yes, and do you know how old the doctor is?" She giggled.

"No, I don't, how old is he?"

"Seventy-three." and she laughed her hearty laugh (so good to hear that again!).

I was amazed that delicate surgery of that degree was still being done by a person of that age, who still had hands steady enough to perform anything near that demanding. I personally knew of three or four surgeons and dentists who had to remove themselves from some or all operative work due to tremors which were more frequent with advancing years. They stopped certain operative procedures, simply because they didn't do enough of them in a year to keep the knife-sharp technique the procedure required.

When I first started in practice it was legal and not uncommon for obstetricians to arrange adoption for those mothers who did not want their babies.

I had a family with eleven children, and the mother was pregnant. Her husband was a laborer, and they lived in a cold water flat. Just being there with their children, you could feel and see the happiness that flowed around that home. One day in the office, she said, "I have asked Dr. Kaplan, my obstetrician, to make arrangements for this baby to be adopted." With this, her eyes filled with tears, which she tried to hide not too successfully from the five-yearold child she had brought in.

"Why are you doing that Helen?" I asked.

"We can't afford any more children. We have our hands full now. Besides, I think it will give him or her better chance in life than we can."

"It is truly a wonderful thing to do, Helen, and I know how very hard this must be for you."

"You have no idea doctor, but I know it's the right thing to do."

When the baby was born, I attended it as I had done for her other kids, and when she went home without her child, a beautiful boy, I bled for her.

I had been told by Dr. Kaplan that the adopting parents would be in the next day and wanted the baby circumcised. The next morning they arrived at nine. The baby was all set to go. I gave them instructions on care of the circumcision and asked them: "Do you have any questions?"

"Yes, doctor. Will you be the baby's doctor?"

"Of course. Please call my office tomorrow and report to the nurse and set up your first appointment."

Neither the adoptive mother nor the biological mother ever met each other, although there were times over the years when they were both in the office at the same time.

The children of both families grew well and were successes in life, but none of the eleven went further than high school, while the adopted boy went through college and became a successful engineer. That would have made Helen proud, but I'm sure also sadness would continue to endure. I wondered how many of the eleven, given the chance their brother had gotten, would have done as well or even better.

Giving away your own flesh and blood, one that you had felt kicking and moving inside you, is without any doubt the most generous gift by that selfless woman that I have ever witnessed.

The call came in the middle of the night. I had twin boys being born whose mother was Rh negative, setting the scene for possible trouble. The Coombs test done at birth was positive, meaning that there was destruction of the boys' red blood cells by antibodies in the mother's blood. Both babies (identical twin boys) were very anemic at birth because of the destruction of their cells, and needed immediate exchange transfusions. But two at once?

One look at their blood counts answered that question, so we cross matched them with compatible Rh negative blood, put the babies side by side on an operating table, and alternated exchanging their blood in 20 cc aliquots. Take 20 cc's out of baby A, discharge it into the waste bucket, then take 20 cc's of his donated Rh negative blood and run it in his umbilical vein. Repeat the process with baby B and his donated blood. Operating thus, I exchanged the two units of blood completely, and then put the babies in incubators under the fluorescent lights to help keep the jaundice from getting too high again.

I went to see the mom. "Well, Marge, Aloysius and Boleslaw (for Baby A and Baby B) are all done. They had their exchange transfusions and should do well. We'll keep checking their Bilirubin levels [the level of jaundice in their blood] in case they need another exchange."

Mom smiled and said, "Aloysius and Boleslaw—I'll bet that will stick!"

And it did. If I see them now around town they'll say, "Hi, Doc! Remember me? I'm Aloysius!" or "Boleslaw!"

PART 10

JIMMY

In February 1968, Jane and I flew out to Aspen with friends, and were looking forward to skiing with them, as well as our son Jim and his friends who were students at the University of Denver and would be with us for the weekend. Jim looked just great and was very happy to be with us. His friends Bogie Hunter and Ron Lyons were good skiers, too. I considered them all experts.

Saturday we decided to ski Snowmass Mountain all day. The boys tried to slow down enough to ski with us, but it just wasn't any fun for them. They could do a trail in three minutes that would take us ten. Finally, I called, "Jim! Why don't you guys go and ski at your own rate and we will meet you at the restaurant at Sam's Knob at one p.m.?"

"Okay, Dad!" Then to Bogie, "I'll race you!" And off they went, with Ron in quick pursuit. As agreed, we met for lunch at Sam's Knob, a restaurant on the mountain- at one, and then parted for the afternoon. We agreed to meet for the five o'clock shuttle, which we all rode back to Aspen together. We adults were sitting around in the living room of our condo having a few snacks and drinks after skiing late afternoon on Saturday. Jim and his friends were out scouting the town. When they arrived at the condo, Jim asked me, "Dad, can I talk to you for a minute?"

"Sure. What's up?"

"Well, I was wondering" Jim started, "there is a ski sale on at the ski store down the street from here, and they have some Red Kneissels on sale for half price. Do you think you could see your way clear to-"

"Say no more Jim. I saw you ski down to the little shed at the bottom of Campground Trail fast as the devil. I saw you ski up the ramp to the roof of that cabin, and jump off the top and ski away with ease. That kind of skiing demands rugged quality equipment. So go ahead and grab them before someone else beats you out of them."

You should have seen his face: huge handsome smile of delight. He and the other two boys were out the door in a flash and returned with the shiny red Kneissels. They were beautiful skis, strong skis, ones that demanded a strong hard skier. They were not recreational skis, but were meant for competition, and he loved them.

Next morning, the seven of us went back to Snowmass and again split up, planning to meet at Sam's Knob for lunch as we had done Saturday. The boys, who were driving back to Denver, wanted to get on the Denver side of the Eisenhower tunnel before nightfall, so we met them at four p.m. to say good bye.

Jane hugged and kissed them all goodbye. Then we loaded our skis on the rack in the back of the shuttle and clambered aboard the bus and took our seats. Jim and his friends watched us board, and as the bus pulled away, Jane waved goodbye and kept waving until I said to her, "Gosh! You'd think you were never going to see him again!"

The rest of our week we skied at Aspen itself on famous seven mile long Ruthie's run, and we also did Aspen Highlands, which boasted the highest chair in the Rockies.

We enjoyed skiing with Didi and Charlie with whom an annual ski trip was a given. We had skied all over the Rockies and in Austria and Switzerland with them as well as many times in Vermont. They were true friends and we enjoyed each others' company.

We returned home on the twenty-first of February and were pleased that Jane's father was coming along satisfactorily. He had been in hospital for a hip replacement, and from all reports, his recovery had been uneventful thus far.

On February twenty eighth I was in the office when my nurse came into the examining room and said, "Excuse me, doctor, but you have an emergency call from Hartford Hospital."

I rushed to my desk. "This is Doctor Rackliffe."

"Doctor, this is the charge nurse on the orthopedic floor. Mr. Baldwin died about twenty minutes ago."

"Jesus! What happened?"

"We think he had a pulmonary embolism. He was in bed feeling fine, and he sat up in bed so that we could freshen him up a bit, and he said, 'I feel funny,' fell back on the pillow, and was gone in a matter of minutes."

I remembered he had had varicose veins, which were frequently the cause of embolisms. The emboli would break off and go to the heart and from there go anywhere, or stay right there in the heart, as it did with Dad Baldwin.

"What would you like me to do?"

"You'll have to come up here and identify him before we can release the body."

"I'll be right up."

I told the staff to cancel the rest of the day and office hours for the next few days and to contact my covering physicians. Then I called Jane and broke the news to her.

"Honey, you go over to your mom's and tell her what's happened. I will meet you there after I am through at Hartford Hospital."

I went up to Hartford and was shown into his room. He looked so peaceful and out of pain. I stayed there for a moment or two with him. Then I gave the hospital officials the name of the undertaker, signed a few papers, and headed for my mother-in-law's house.

As expected, Mother Baldwin was in a pretty bad state because he had been doing so well that this was a complete shock. Thankfully, her two daughters were there with her.

The undertaker wanted some of Dad's clothes brought down to the funeral home. I knew just the outfit that I had always liked on him. I selected his beige gabardine trousers, a dark brown sport coat; a black and white hounds tooth wool shirt, and his favorite Navaho bolo with a silver clasp and brown loafers. He had always looked great in that outfit.

Later, Mother Baldwin asked me to call the vet who was taking care of his hunting dog Tip and have him put down.

As cruel as this sounds, it wasn't. First of all, Tip was over ten years old and he had been raised by Dad Baldwin and handled only by him. He was a trained bird dog and lived only to hunt with his master. No one was allowed to touch him except Dad. He was never allowed in the house. He had a pen in the yard, and whenever he was out of it he was with his owner. Dad used to say that his family had spoiled all his hunting dogs and it wasn't going to happen to this one.

It seemed appropriate that they go on together, and it felt right to issue that order, which was carried out that day. I had a mental picture of them walking towards a golden field with Tip gamboling around in front of him, tail wagging like mad, and Jim with his shotgun cradled comfortably in his arm. What could be better for them?

For the next few days there was a constant line of men and women in their beautiful home, whose construction Dad had lovingly overseen all through, making sure that everything was done exactly to his and her desire. It was a one-floor house that nestled above the twelfth green of the Shuttle Meadow Country Club. The master bedroom and bath spanned the entire southern end of the home. In the hallway leading to the living room was dad's den fitted with cherry cabinets for his guns, fishing rods, and books, with an outdoor porch overlooking the golf course. There was a guest room across the hall from the den, with its own bath.

The hall from the bedrooms emptied into a huge living room. A full width window wall faced the golf course, on the rear side of the house. On a cherry wood-paneled wall that lead from the window to the hallway, there was a Bolton stone fireplace with a raised hearth. The kitchen, dining room, and breakfast room all were entered from the main hallway, at the end of which were stairs down to the recreation room.

This room was under the living room and of equal size. It had a wet bar at one end, and at the other end another Bolton stone fireplace with a raised hearth.

There was a lavatory and an entranceway to the back yard.

This was the room where we celebrated Christmas and thanksgiving every year.

The church service was plain and straightforward, just like the man. It was mostly attended by local company executives and their wives, resplendent in their furs. The service was short, and at the end of the service all the guests were invited back to Shuttle Meadow Country club for hors d'oeuvres and drinks.

In the days that followed the burial, my wife and her sister were a constant presence for their mom; they cried with her and held her close and grieved together.

I reopened my office on the fifth of March, spending time with Mother Baldwin as I could. She wanted a new car, so I took care of that for her.

About ten a.m. on the eighth of March, my secretary called me out of an examining room. "You have an emergency call from New Mexico." I went to my desk to answer the phone thinking, *This has to be Jim.* I put it on speaker phone since it was closer to me, so both of my girls and even some patients heard the conversation.

"Hello?"

" Is this Dr. Rackliffe, father of James P. Rackliffe?"

I thought, *Oh boy, probably broke a leg or something.* "Yes, it is."

"This is the administrator of the Tularosa New Mexico General Hospital speaking. Your son was brought in here this morning dead on arrival."

I fell into my chair in disbelief, overwhelmed and unable to think. Linda and Pat—my office staff—jumped to the phone, and after telling them what funeral home to send my son—my son!—I thought, *what do I do now?*

Jane - I had to find her. She was probably at her mother's home. There was no answer at our house, so I headed for her mother's home. When I got there, I rang the bell. Jane opened the door, and I blurted out "Jane, it's Jimmy." From the look on my face, she knew immediately, and so did her mother who immediately became the comforter instead of the comforted.

We went home and had the boys released from school. Dan and Peter took the news surprisingly well—I don't recall either of them crying, but I'm sure they did. Steve, who was Jimmy's roommate and only twelve, cried and cried inconsolably and kept asking, "Why?"

I couldn't answer him. I remembered how beautiful a skier Jim was and how gracious he looked, or if racing, how determined.

I remembered one day watching Jim come down the fairway with a golf bag on each shoulder, complimenting his players to get a bigger tip, a huge grin on his face; I remember him and his best friend Bill Bray when camping in the Thousand Islands, trying to impress a couple of young American girls by speaking with Canadian accents. I remembered when he was two, wearing matching swim trunks on the beach at Meigs Point. Jane had made them for us. I remember taking him out in my arms and swimming along with him,- hand firmly under that tender little tummy while he was doing the dog paddle. I remembered how at age two, he took a shower with me and took hold of the nearest support - my penis—how that made me laugh. Oh Jim! Never again. Never again. No more four boy "pig piles on Dad" in the living room; no more racing down to the recreation room on Christmas mornings. I felt as though a huge piece of me was missing—just ripped right out of me.

Reverend Alan MacLean was a life saver for Steve. He spent almost all his day helping Steve cope. Jim had been Steve's hero. losing your favorite person is hard at any age, but especially so in the late preteen years.

Jane, poor woman, losing her father and son in a ten-day span, spent a lot of time in the woods - just sitting. It had to be a terrible burden. It was tough for me; it must have been an absolute nightmare for her. Strangely though, we never went to each other and embraced, as I had seen many parents do over this huge loss.

Jim's body did not arrive here until Monday due to bad weather. We had a private viewing with my brother Foster and his wife Marie. Jimmy looked like he was sleeping. Not a mark on him, thank God.

We did not bring his brothers to see him for the last time on earth because we felt it would make it even harder than it was, especially for Stevie. Jane and I were glad that my brother Foster and his wife Marie were with us in that dark somber room.

Even in death he looked so young, so handsome-gone forever. If only I could have changed places with him, it would have been the way it's supposed to be.

Since there were no calling hours, the house was full of people and family trying to show their sorrow at our loss. Some of my patients came to the door with food. I remember opening the door and there was one of my moms - a black lady named Rose Hill standing there with lasagna. I burst into tears when I saw her, and she said, "Stop your blubbering man, this is going to taste good!" She handed it to me and turned and left. She didn't want to let her sorrow show, but I knew her, and understood her quick departure.

All that time between the news of his death on Thursday through Monday when his body finally got home there was constant activity: flowers, people, food, and even liquor were being brought in with all of our friends coming to be with us and help us through this horrible time. They were quiet around us but there were conversations going in all corners of the house. I saw to it that those who wanted drinks got them and talked about Jim to anyone who brought it up.

"How did it happen Bob? Why New Mexico? I thought he was in school at the University of Denver."

"I have not heard a word from the University, which I think is pretty awful. Apparently the four kids were on their way to Mexico for some reason. Ron West, Jim's friend, talked Jim into going at the last minute. So the four of them took off, with a guy from New York driving a car registered in Oregon and loaned to them by the owner's daughter. On the outskirts of Tularosa at eighty miles per hour they hit a tractor trailer full of oranges weighing thirty tons, head on. Two were killed instantly, the driver suffered severe head injuries, and Ron West walked away uninjured. The truck driver, a woman, was not hurt either."

"Well, Bob, I'm sorry, and if there is anything I can do, just call."

"Thanks, Bill."

Mark and Bill Jones had opened their clothing store in order to measure and fit Dan, Peter, and Steve with clothes for the funeral. None of them had a suit, so they needed to be fitted with suits, shirts, shoes and ties. They looked nice, but for the wrong reason.

The day of the funeral, I awoke early to the sound of mourning doves (how appropriate). It was a gray damp day, perfect for the sadness that would attend us all that day.

As we walked out of the house, down the flagstones walk past the brown grass to the waiting limousine, I had the strangest feeling that this was all false and that we were on stage acting out a macabre play.

Jane, Dan, and I sat in the rear seat, and Peter and Steve sat in the jump seats in front of us. As the car backed out of the driveway and turned to go down the street, there was silence. There was not one word spoken all the way to the church by anyone. We were all dealing with the thoughts in our own heads, bewildered that such an occasion was taking place, that Jim would never be with us again.

When we arrived at the side door of the church, Rev. Alan MacLean met us, and as we prepared to go into the side door of the church, Father Ed McLean came rushing out of a parking lot across the street and extended his hand to Rev. Alan.

"I'm Father McLean, and I am going to take part in Jim's service."

He was welcomed by Alan (Reverend MacLean) who said, "Thank you very much for coming Father, both the family and I will be honored to have you taking part in the service."

Father Ed had driven down from Stowe, Vermont, that morning to be there for Jim. We had skied with Father Ed many times, but to hear he had come all that way for our Jimmy brought fourth another round of tears from Jane and me.

The family was ushered in to a side room in the front of the church on the left side of the altar. At the appropriate moment, we were to enter the church as a family. When the door opened and we were motioned into the front pews of the church, I gasped.

This huge old gothic brownstone church, with its superb Cooper pipe and echo organs, had a balcony so that the seating capacity was about 1,200, and it was packed with students. The high school had a student body of about 3,000. Jim had been very well known and liked, so the kids told their teachers they were going to his funeral - period. They filled the church.

Once again, I was awash in tears. The service was a blur to me, and the procession to the Palmer/Baldwin plot in Fairview Cemetery occurred without any memory to me. I do remember walking over the grass to a freshly dug hole ready to receive and keep my son for eternity. That was an ugly thought, too.

Many came back to the house for drinks and food (all planned for and prepared by Jane Sweeney and Didi Goldstein). it was subdued but not unpleasant. There was small talk and laughter, drinks and food (a lot of which had been prepared and brought over by friends and neighbors). Finally the last guest or family member had left. We were alone, and it was over.

I will never forget Jane Sweeney and Didi. They practically moved in for a week and ran the house. When I took Jane home the last time, and tried to thank her, she started to cry and said, "You saved my Tommy, don't ever forget that."

Finally Jane and I were alone. We sat in quiet contemplation and the only sound was the chiming of the grandfather's clock and the quiet sounds coming from the boys' rooms upstairs.

PART 11:

LIFE AFTER JIM

The week following his burial brought forth its own demons with which we were forced to deal:

1. Disbelief: We would sleep and dream that the whole thing was just a dream only to wake up to the grim reality. Or we wouldn't sleep at all. Both of us lived through the terror of the oncoming truck full of oranges, shouting to Jim, "Look out!" The yard seemed full of mourning doves who kept at it all day long. To this day, they bring back memories of Jim whenever I hear their melancholy song.

I'm sure that we both had these moments of bad dreams and sad thoughts, but we never discussed them with each other.

2. Flowers: The arrival of flowers on the day he was killed continued even after he was buried. During the time from his death until his body arrived in New Britain (five days), we were deluged with bouquets, and the smell of flowers permeated the house. The aroma was

so overpowering it made me feel nauseated. Whenever the doorbell rang and more flowers were presented, it was hard to say, "Thank you."

About two weeks after the funeral we began to receive a few more flowers, and I noticed that in these late arrivals the senders had one thing in common. They had all been through the loss of a family member, and those flowers were accepted gratefully by us. After that experience, we always waited two weeks to send a floral arrangement to someone who was grieving.

3. Anger: I had seen it in survivors of patients who had died. Now I felt it! I was angry - damned angry! Who was the son of a bitch driving that fucking car at eighty mph right into a truck load of oranges. Damn him! Why hadn't he died And Ron West, the kid who talked my son into going, how dare he walk away unscathed!

And why were they going to Tijuana, Mexico? I have an idea as to the reason for that trip, but I'd rather just leave the question unanswered.

I wrote a letter, that fairly burned, to the president of Denver University, castigating him for his lack of caring, for not even calling or writing us about our son's death! Outrageous! If we had depended on this Ph.D. person to notify us about the death of one of his students, who happened to be my son, who knows when we would have heard? His pusillanimous response further enraged me:

"The girl who was killed was from a dear family that we know very well, and I was so saddened by it that I spent most of my time with the bereaved family. I just left my office and University affairs to my staff, and went to them. I realize now that this was wrong, and I apologize."

Incompetent ass!

I called Bill McQueeney, a lawyer friend of mine and told him I wanted to sue the driver of the car, but the suit ended up being against the Oregon owner of the car, who wasn't in the picture at all. Bill started the lawsuit, which was going to take a long time to get to court, due to the complexity of the case, a New York driver in a car registered in Oregon, causing two fatalities in New Mexico.

After about two weeks, a truck from a local garden shop arrived with a beautiful Star Magnolia tree that the delivery man planted it for us. It was a gift from a psychiatrist in town with this unwritten message: "Look upon the beautiful things in life and enjoy them." It didn't say that in writing -it just was beautiful and living, and it affected both Jane and me deeply, as the blossoms moved slowly in the breeze. We had it planted outside the kitchen window where we could see the star-shaped bracts every day that it was in bloom.

When Jim's stuff came from Denver, complete with the red Kneissels, there was a raincoat in Jim's luggage. The raincoat belonged to Arute Brothers Contractors where he had worked as summer help.

Jimmy had come home one day wearing one of these raincoats, and it was a beauty! It was a thigh-length rubberized yellow coat with a corduroy collar. Written across the back of the coat in five-inch letters was "ARUTE BROS.CO".

I made the comment upon seeing it, "That's a good looking coat for rough weather."

Jimmy nodded and said, "It's really cool. I think I'll take it when I go to Denver."

"No, Jim. You can't do that. That's stealing, and besides Mr. Arute is a friend of mine."

Here it was in his luggage, which Bogie and several of his other friends packed up and shipped at their expense. I immediately took it down to Jack Arute, whose children were under my care.

When he saw me coming, he rushed out the door, threw the rain jacket over his shoulder, and took me out to lunch. I wasn't making much sense, so after we parted he called one of my partners, expressing his concern. Dr. Vinnie Ringrose, a good friend, came over to the house, and with his help and Charlie's (my skiing buddy), they helped me find a level place to stand, as my whole world had fallen apart. Charlie hit home when he said, "Bob, you just need time."

And he was right. The only thing that softens a loss like that is time. I got to the point in a few weeks that when people expressed regrets, I could thank them without tearing up.

About a week to ten days after the funeral, I found myself going over to Jim's grave a lot at noon and just sitting there. One day, there was a single rose on his grave and it filled me with curiosity. Who left it? Was it a girl who had secretly mourned for him? Was it the one he had left when he went to Denver? I would never know, but she would have been my first bet.

Jim's death taught me how a human being reacts to the death of a loved one. It made me a better doctor. I understood the disbelief, the sorrow, the anger, and the desire to strike back that I had seen with my parents when they lost a child, because I went through all those emotions.

About a year after our loss, I was asked to speak to a group at the University, a support group for people who were grieving. The purpose of this group was to have people dealing with tragedies meet and listen to others and get support from them or the moderator. We sat in a circle of about fourteen persons, and I told my story first, then we went round the circle as each one spoke. At the end, I commented on each couples' loss, sympathized with them, reassured them they were recovering, and told them to stay the course as they were doing. There were two instances where I felt I had to speak differently to the parent or parents.

The first was a young lady who was there alone, and she wept the entire evening.

"Michelle," I said when I got to her, "would you like to tell us your story?"

Michelle's lip quivered, and through her tears she said, "I lost Peter, my two- month old son, one month ago from SIDS." She burst into tears again. "I can't stop crying! When will it stop?"

I answered her quietly. "You shouldn't even be here, Michelle. It's too early for you to be here. *You should be crying*—that's normal for this time in your loss, so go home and cry. I promise you, with the passage of time, it will get better."

The other couple that concerned me was the Andersons, who said, "We lost our son in an automobile accident, just like you did, doctor."

"How long has it been since you lost him?"

"It's been eighteen years."

I said, "I am very sorry for your loss, and you have a perfect right to think of him, and at times, feel sad, but it's been eighteen years! It's time for you to put that grief behind you, and to start making an attempt to live your life happily, with new interests and friends, and get back to the living. You should not come to these grieving sessions, as you are just prolonging your sorrow. You must get over that and go on with life. Thank God you have each other."

In a few weeks, I was back to full practice, seeing my usual forty-five to fifty-five children per day in the office. At home things were getting back to normal, and, as the weather warmed, Jane and I resumed playing golf together evenings during the week, and weekends with other couples. The first time back however, we went out alone on a Sunday afternoon, and everyone respected our privacy.

In the late 1950s, a new addition to the hospital was in the works, one with seven operating suites on the ground floor, with the original plan calling for a new three-story central building. At the time, there was a very savvy chairman of the board of directors running the show. (They were always local businessmen who would serve two years, and sometimes more.) This chairman made a canny observation to the effect that it would cost far less to erect four floors, and leave the unused one empty 'til needed. While there was no plumbing, only sparse electricity, and no rooms, the in-wall pipes and outlets were in place. It was just a cavernous concrete place, with nothing in it except the barest essentials that could be finished and functional in a heart beat. It was an ugly concrete place, but in an emergency, it could be useable in a matter of hours. It was all just sitting there empty in late May of 1962.

During that month, the Berlin High School sponsored a Roman style meal, and every one of the students was supposed to come to the meal in a toga. Most of them ate some of the potato salad. Almost immediately after the meal, masses of students headed for bathrooms and outdoors, vomiting and cramping with diarrhea. They flowed into the neighborhood, some collapsing on lawns, some making it further than others before collapsing. People driving by started picking them up, as did the local police, and started transporting them to the hospital, to the woefully inadequate emergency room. This had originally been the hospital operating room, with another four rooms that were much smaller. Into this small space came better than one hundred ten or so vomiting adolescents, many of whom were also having diarrhea. In less than one hour there was at least a half inch of vomitus on the floor of the entire emergency room.

Doctors who were not working that day (one of whom was me) were summoned to help out. What a scene to be confronted with when I arrived at the ER. Automobile after automobile drove up to unload another toga-clad student, many of whom could barely walk. Others were put on gurneys and wheeled into the ER, vomiting as they went.

Rapidly, the unused new floor was the focus of attention. I went up to that floor to start assessing and treating the young and very sick patients.

Beds with mattresses were being put together by one batch of workers of the maintenance crew. Following right behind them, nurses and nurses' aides made the beds, and then lifted a waiting patient into it. The four doctors, each with a nurse, were following down four lanes of beds, examining each patient as soon as they got into a bed. We were starting IVs to rehydrate them. We gave those who were vomiting a shot of medicine to get that under control.

Another group of maintenance men connected bed pan washers, and a flush basin was hooked up. The number of lights was tripled and a phone was connected.

As the patients were triaged through the ER, some got a shot and went home, but eighty-five were sent up to our quickly filling floor. Students were lined up on gurneys waiting for beds, but the wait for treatment became less and less as the team of workers on that floor worked smoothly along, in an increasingly capable and friendly atmosphere of cooperation. Bed pans were in use big time. Since there had been no time or plan to separate by sex, and there were no drapes around the beds, the patients just looked the other way when their neighbor had a problem.

Within three hours, this empty floor had eighty-five patients, lights, running water, a phone, nurses, and doctors, and all was settling down. Many of the patients were sleeping, physically and emotionally drained.

I was so proud of those kids! The way they respected each other's privacy was just great. I was also proud to be part of that group who had responded to the challenge so magnificently.

Thank God the extra unused floor had been built.

One night after an especially long and busy day, I came home to a dark house. Emptying the mail box of a large amount of mail, I entered the back hall and threw the pile of mail on the kitchen table. Jane was on one of her golf trips, so I was living alone for a few days.

I looked at the mail on the table, and on the top of the pile was a card from the Klingberg Children's Home announcing a special meeting about the Tucson property. Lying next to it was *TIME* magazine, conveniently opened to an article entitled, "Boom in the Southwest." During dinner, I read the article about the area, especially about Tucson. Everything was flourishing there, and the city was growing like moss on wet soil. *Hmmm*, I thought.

The night of the meeting I took the magazine with me. A lawyer on the board had flown out to Tucson to appraise the situation. Our land was a sixty-acre piece of land donated to the home after the article about Rev. Klingberg had appeared in *Reader's Digest* in 1943.

The lawyer said, "Our land is bordered on two sides by interstate highway, and we have been offered $350,000 for it. My recommendation to the board is to accept the offer."

I remembered our last real estate transaction when we sold a piece of land for $40,000, which was recouped by the buyer who sold the top soil for that, and then sold the land in several parts making another $175,000 in the process. If it hadn't been for *TIME magazine* being open to that part, I wouldn't have known enough to suggest that we might do better.

With the magazine article on the table in front of me, I raised my hand, and Don (who had taken over managing the home in1968, thus starting the third generation of Klingbergs) recognized me.

"I want to thank John for going out to Tucson and evaluating the situation firsthand," I said, "However, when I got home last Thursday announcing this meeting, lying on the table was *Time* magazine open to the article entitled, 'Boom in the Southwest' that caught my eye. Since our land is bordered on two sides by interstate highways, and the city is growing in our direction, I would think that we should hold on to it for the time being. After all, the taxes are only $500 per year, so I think we should wait for a better offer."

After some discussion, the decision was made to reject the offer and hold on to the land.

Within two years, it was sold for over one million dollars.

I think it was divine providence that the magazine fell open to that article.

Early one morning as I was getting ready for work, the answering service called;

"Dr. Rackliffe? Mrs. Meyer is on the phone and has an emergency. May I patch her through?"

"Yes, of course. … Mrs. Meyer? This is Doctor Rackliffe. What is the matter?"

"Oh, Doctor, thank you for answering. Theresa choked on some peanuts that she found in the living room an hour ago, and she hasn't stopped coughing since. I'm so worried about her, doctor."

"She probably has one in her lung, Mrs. Meyer. Please take her up to the hospital, and I will take care of things. I'll see you up there."

"Thank you, Doctor; we will go up right now."

I then called the ER and alerted them to a 4 year old patient of mine coming in, and ordered a chest x-ray to be done immediately on arrival. Fluoroscopy was to be done as soon as a radiologist came in.

After seeing her and listening to her chest, there was no doubt that she had indeed aspirated a peanut. The fact that it was a peanut was worrisome, since the oil in the peanut was especially dangerous because of the pneumonia it caused. I knew of one little boy who had died after aspirating one. I alerted our bronchcoscopist on staff, and he booked her immediately for general anesthesia so that he could get a good thorough look.

After he examined her in the operating room under anesthesia, he called me.

"Bob? This is Len. Your girl is in recovery room. I couldn't find anything."

Great! Now what? I decided to send her home on antibiotics and check with the mom the next morning. My call that morning to Mrs. Meyer was not good.

"She coughed all night, doctor, and now she is so tired from coughing."

"Well I think we still have a peanut in there, Mrs. Meyer. Let's take her up to Hartford Hospital and have their bronchcoscopist take a look. I'll make the arrangements."

I called the ER at Hartford Hospital, and told the doc about my problem case that was on her way up there, and asked that he call in their best bronchoscopist. Once again, Theresa was put under general anesthesia and bronchoscoped with the same result: No foreign body found.

I knew there was a peanut in there because of the way she breathed on fluoroscopic exam, so I decided to send her down to New York City to be seen at Manhattan Eye and Ear Hospital, and I made the arrangements for her to go there the next morning.

About six hours after she had left for New York, I got a phone call.

"Please hold for Dr. Rabbit."

In about two minutes a cheery voice came on. "Hi, Dr. Rackliffe. This is Tom Rabbit. I saw your girl in the ER this morning, sprayed her throat with a little topical anesthesia, and took out the peanut. She did fine, and is on her way home."

"You did it in the ER?" (I couldn't believe it.)

"Yep. Nothing to it. By the way, what does her father do?

"He works in a factory."

Dr. Rabbit's bill was $200.

About a year of two after that, I had another child who aspirated part of a carrot stick. This time, I sent her directly to Manhattan Eye and Ear Hospital after calling them to alert them to her arrival.

Similar to the last time, in about six hours Dr. Rabbit was on the phone, and just like the last time, the carrot stick was removed in the ER with only topical anesthesia.

"They're on their way home now, Dr. Rackliffe."

"You're amazing, Dr. Rabbit. How many of these cases do you do?"

"That's all I do every day, all year. By the way, what does this father do?"

"He's president of the local national bank."

Dr. Rabbit's bill was $2,000.

Every morning I would start my hospital rounds in the nursery, checking all my babies. One morning I had one new one, a baby boy named D'Agostino weighed seven pounds, and who looked just great. There was nothing at all worrisome about him.

After seeing the babies, I started on rounds to talk to the mothers. When I entered Mrs. D'Agostino's room, she was sitting straight up and was dressed like a queen with a satin jacket over a very lovely night gown.

"Hello, Mrs. D'Agostino. I am Dr. Rackliffe, and I will be taking care of your baby."

"I'ma glada to meet you, Doc. Howsa my boy Giuseppe?" She smiled proudly.

"He's just fine. He weighs seven pounds. Are you going to breast feed him?"

"No, doc. I don't a wanta do that."

"Okay. We'll put him on formula then, but don't worry if he doesn't eat in the first few days. Babies never do. I'll see you again tomorrow morning then. By the way, do you want him circumcised?" (I knew the answer to that one. She was just over from the old country, and it was never done there because the Nazis had called every circumcised male Jewish during WWII.)

"No doc, don'ta cut."

At the office about three hours later a call came from the nursery, asking to speak to me.

"Hi, this is Dr. Rackliffe. What's up?"

"It's the D'Agostino baby, doctor. He's getting very jaundiced, so we ordered some blood tests that we knew you would want. They don't look too good. His bilirubin (at 15 hours) was 16. His blood type is AB + and his mother is O+. The Rh test is negative."

"It looks like an ABO incompatibility, and we are heading for trouble. Thank you for doing the lab tests. Please order a cross match for a unit of O negative blood and repeat the bilirubin at twelve noon."

"Yes, doctor."

Somewhere in the past, this mother had been transfused with AB blood, and had manufactured antibodies to those genes that were now destroying her son's blood at a prodigious rate.

The noon bilirubin was pushing 20 mgm%, so I set up to do an exchange transfusion. while the operating room was being prepared, I went in to see Mrs. D'Agostino.

"Mrs. D'Agostino, we have a problem. Giuseppe needs to have a transfusion because his blood cells are different than yours and are being destroyed."

"He's *a morte*!" she cried, and started saying it over and over again.

"He's not *a morte*!" I reassured her. "I just have to exchange his blood, so don't worry, and I'll be back in about an hour and a half."

"He's *a morte*!" she cried, as I left for surgery.

The exchange went smoothly and I brought him in to show him to Mrs. D'Agostino about six p.m. She was all smiles.

Twelve midnight that night I was back, and woke Mrs. D'Agostino. "Mrs. D'Agostino, Giuseppe needs another exchange. His yellow color is getting bad again, so I am going to arrange another exchange transfusion right now."

That tipped off another round of "He's *a morte*!" and a lot of crying and moaning, but by one-thirty, Giuseppe was back in his mother's arms again and Mrs. D'Agostino was all smiles again.

At five a.m., we went through this scenario for the third time. We were gaining ground though, because Giuseppe made it for twelve hours to the next exchange. At that time we went back for round four, and again, Mrs. D'Agostino reassured me for the twenty-third time that Giuseppe was a cooked goose."He's *a morte*, doctor, he's *a morte*!"

When the "He's *a morte*!" chant started again, I turned and looked down at her and said firmly and loudly: "Giuseppe is not *a morte*! He wouldn't dare! He's got Polack blood, Yankee blood,and Jewish blood, German blood, and Swedish blood in his veins, and with all that good stuff, he wouldn't dare *a morte* He's a notta going to *morte*, damn it!"

During the next two days he was obviously cured, and the day before discharge I went in to see her, as she had him sleeping in the crook of her arm.

"You know, Doctor, I been a thinkin. Giuseppe was-a born on St. Martin's-a day, so Im a gonna name-a him, Giuseppe Martino D'Agostino."

"No, Mrs. D'Agostino, you are NOT. You are going to name him Giuseppe Martino Roberto D'Agostino," I responded. "After all the time I have spent up here with Giuseppe, he's a little bit mine now, so I want my name on him, too. Okay?"

She looked up at me and smiled: "That'sa nice a name. I'ma gonna do it."

So she did, but I never heard from her again. She moved back to Italy and after a year or so, I got a letter from an Italian physician written in Italian that she was pregnant, and please tell him about the first pregnancy, specifically about the baby, including diagnosis and treatment. I found a person who could write Italian, and we sent a lengthy letter explaining the problem and what to do about it. She went on to deliver a live baby again, but sadly, the doctor wrote us that "he's *a morte*" a few days after birth.

On December 23, 1968, I made a house call to Mrs. Mulligan's home. She lived in one of the low income projects left over from the housing built for factory workers in World War II. She wanted me to see her daughter Mary, who had "been sick for a few days with a high fever and a cough." Because I suspected a bacterial infection, possibly pneumonia, I brought along enough samples of medicine to spare them the cost if it were needed.

Mrs. Mulligan, a tall thin woman, greeted me at the door. "Thank you for coming, doctor. Please come in, and excuse the way the kitchen looks. With Mary sick, I've kind of let things slide here."

The kitchen floor was a patchwork of linoleum pieces that overlaid each other. There was a small old refrigerator. In the corner next to it stood a scrawny Christmas tree. Hanging from every available vestige of a branch were home made decorations the children must have made.

There were three or four unmistakable little Irish faces, complete with freckles, standing around the dilapidated, curtain-less kitchen, examining me and my bag. "Mary is upstairs, Doctor, and she is wearing her Christmas present so you could see it."

Her christmas present - as in one! And I thought of the obscene number of gifts my boys were getting.

I climbed the worn stairs to a dimly lighted dingy hallway, and proceeded across to a room with two sets of steel bunk beds, one set on each wall. A light bulb with an old fabric shade hung from the center of the ceiling. There was one steel double window with cranks to open them, partially covered by a torn, stained shade. There was no closet, and a chest of five drawers was the only furniture other than the wooden chair Mrs. Mulligan offered to me.

In the lower right hand bunk, Mary lay with a smile that an angel carried to her from heaven for that moment. She was wearing her Christmas present: a red and white candy-striped flannel night gown, which was accentuated by her fevered bright red cheeks and startlingly blue eyes.

She was beautiful! She just glowed so that the room no longer looked drab, but radiated the beauty of the child.

"Hi, Mary," I said. "How are you feeling?" Her temperature was 104 degrees.

"Fine thank you, doctor," she coughed, and a look of pain came over her face and erased her smile for a fraction of time but then it returned, even more angelic and beautiful than before.

"I think your Christmas present is almost as beautiful as you are." I said.

She smiled.

"Would you mind sitting up for me? I would like to listen to your back."

I helped her to sit up, opened the buttons on the top of the nightshirt and after warning her, "This'll be cold!" slid my stethoscope down inside her nightshirt on her back. This produced a monumental case of "goose pimples."

After listening to her chest, it was, as I had feared, a raging pneumonia in her right lower lobe in the back. I gave her a pat and said, "Mary, you have a cold in your lungs, and I am going to have to give you an injection. This will hurt a little bit, but if you say the magic words, 'Suffering Succotash!' when I say, 'Go,' it won't be too bad. Okay?"

"Okay, doctor."

"Fine. Now you roll over onto your stomach, and I'll tell you when to say the magic words." I pulled up her night shirt exposing her white little bottom, and after preparing the injection, was ready to go. "Okay, Mary, go!"

"Suffering Succotash—ow!"

I rubbed the spot for a minute with an alcohol swab, and then said, "Great job Mary! You are all fixed! Did it hurt too much?"

"No, doctor, it wasn't bad."

"Well now, we'll have you up and around by Christmas day, young lady, and I have to thank you for letting me see you in your beautiful Christmas present!"

I helped the exhausted child to turn over and went back down stairs.

"Mary has pneumonia, Mrs. Mulligan, but I have brought some medicine with me, because I feared that was the case after talking with you."

Mrs. Mulligan took the medicine from me and when she opened the refrigerator to put it away, I could see the shelves were bare, except for a bottle of milk.

"I'll call you in the morning to see how she's doing." I said as I opened the door to leave.

When I got back to my car I was thinking: *Some Christmas: A night gown for her only present and no food in the house!* When I got back to the office I called Don Klingberg at the Children's Home and told him the whole story. Then I asked him, "Do you guys get a lot of stuff at Christmas time, like toys, clothes, and food?"

"We always do, Bob. Just give me the names and ages of the children, and we'll send over clothes, toys, and food, like a turkey, a bag of potatoes, some vegetables and fruit, and a fruitcake, too. We're getting a lot of those this year."

On December 24, Mary was better, and a huge delivery of gifts from the Children's Home arrived midday with all the promised goods, much to the delight of the little Mulligans.

At that time I had been taking care of the Mulligans for about four years, and after that visit, I never saw them again, until one day, about two years later, I bumped into Mrs. Mulligan in a downtown store.

"Hello, Mrs. Mulligan! Long time no see! How are you and the kids?

"Fine, doctor, thank you."

"Tell me Mrs. Mulligan, why did you leave me? I've missed not seeing you."

"Well you know, doctor, we never paid you, and because you had done so much for us, we felt it was time to give someone else a try, to be fair to you."

I really missed that family.

PART 12:

CAMPING ON THE VINEYARD

J ane and I were sitting in the kitchen having breakfast on a spring morning. We were discussing summer plans after the loss of Jimmy.

"I don't think we will be camping this year, will we?" she asked.

"Of course, we're going camping!" I replied, "Not only that, but each boy is going to bring a friend."

When I told our friend Betty Eddy about our plans to go camping and to take three extra boys with us she said, "Wonderful! Why don't you spend one week with us on the Vineyard? There is plenty of room for you to camp on our land." I knew that the Eddy family owned a lot of land on Martha's Vineyard, and it sounded like a perfect spot.

"Thank you, Betty. That sounds great! Are your sure you're up to having six teenage boys romping around here for a week?"

"It'll be fun," she replied, "I'm sure Bud will have them all working for him before the week is out." Bud was her husband, and he had built the house we were going to visit himself. He was a man's man, a graduate of Yale (as all the males in the family were for generations). He had his own business, was very creative, and showed a great love of life. He would be fun to be around.

When I got home and told Jane about the invitation, she was pleased and excited about the prospect, too.

"Well that takes care of one week. I've been looking at the campgrounds along the New Jersey shore, and there is one in Wildwood that sounds pretty nice. It is right on the water. We could go there for the second week, after we stop at home to change kids, if there are any changes. Do you think the boys would like to take other friends on the second week?"

"I don't know. Why don't we let them make that decision?"

The boys were delighted at the plans. Dan had Kim Bray for the first week and Carl Zimmerman for the second. Peter and Steve each took one friend for the entire two weeks.

The trip to Martha's Vineyard came first. On a beautiful warm morning, we packed six boys and Jane and me into the Dodge station wagon with the camper (aka "baby") attached behind, and took off for the Vineyard ferry. About four hours later, we were on a very narrow black top road heading for the Eddys, who lived in Chilmark. After a sharp turn towards the sea and up a modest hill, we saw a house on the right that fit the description. "There's an oil drum astride the roof." Just before the house, was a driveway with a crude sign facing us: "Welcome to Resurrection City!"

We drove in the dirt and stone driveway level to the back of the house, where we could easily see the oil drum straddling the roof with a pipe trailing down the rear of the house and heading towards the driveway.

Out the rear door came Betty and her youngest daughter Susie, rushing towards us. "Well here you are! Thank heavens! The directions must have been right for a change."

Hers was a voice with a built-in smile.

"Now, you have a choice. You can sleep in the boat-house, which has been converted to a guest house and sleeps six, but you could squeeze in eight if you wanted. It has running water and a bathroom. Or you can set up your tent and use both."

At this point, her husband Bud came around the corner of the house and joined us. Pointing up to the top of a hill behind the boat house he said: "You could put your tent up there."

Between "there" and where we sat there was a thick cover of small trees and brush, some with trunks of one and a half inches or more.

"How do I get up there?"

"Just drive right up through the bush." he replied.

"I don't think I could make it up there."

"Sure you can. Watch." Saying that, he strode to his Pontiac station wagon started the engine, put it in gear and plowed right up the hill through all the trees and brush until he reached the top. Then he turned the car around and came right back down to us.

"See?" He smiled.

"Okay. If you can do it, I sure as hell can try." I slipped behind the wheel, put the car in low gear, and attacked with no intention of stopping 'til I had equaled his mark, trailer notwithstanding.

The Dodge made it with ease, and "baby" came along without a problem.

The Eddys said they would see us at cocktail hour or earlier if we needed anything, and left us to settle in.

Dan, Kim, Peter, and Buden elected to stay in the boat house, while "Finner" (Bob Finn) and Steve chose to stay with us in the tent. The site was the highest hill for miles, and there was a magnificent view of the island and the Atlantic Ocean from there. It was exposed to the breezes, and parts of the tent flapped in the wind.

Having decided that meals would be at the boat-house, we did not put up the tarpaulin and picnic table. Only the aluminum framed tent and trailer were up on the top of the hill.

When we joined the Eddys for cocktails, Bud said to the boys, "I'm going back to the city for the week, so I want to show you fellows how to get the water to the roof drum, because you are going to be responsible for it all week." He started back down towards the driveway, with all the boys following, and me tagging along, too. Across the driveway there was a little stream gurgling away down the hill. Bud had made the stream deeper in one area and had a gasoline engine-driven pump there with the pump submerged. He showed the boys how to start it, and then said, "When you see water running down the roof, turn it off."

How ingenious!

Jane and I joined the Eddys for cocktails, while the boys made some supper at the boathouse. The Eddys' dog Patches, a black and white English Cocker Spaniel, enjoyed all the company, and he was a hoot to watch. When he wagged his tail, his whole rear end wagged. If he were chasing his ball after it had been thrown, he would literally jump up with all four legs in the air to get a better look. Jane and I fell in love with the little fella.

After supper of hot dogs and beans, we chatted a while, and eventually everyone went to bed. About two hours later we awoke to hear a coming storm. The lightning was all around the island, striking the sea as it approached. Jane and Finner left for the boat house.

"Aren't you coming?" she asked me.

"No, this is perfectly safe here, we're grounded."

Steve elected to stay with me.

"I think that's very dangerous. I wish you would come with us," she said as the thunder and lightning increased in intensity.

Old stubborn and his innocent son stayed put in the "safe" grounded tent on the top of the hill.

It was the wildest night of my life since the bombings of Saipan. Gale force winds were driving sheets of rain at us horizontally; the thunder and lightning were almost continuous and lasted for hours. Steve and I stayed in the double bed in the center of the tent on the trailer.

Finally, it was over. The next morning Betty stood on the rear porch of her house and called over: "Are you all right?"

"Yes, thank you, but tell me, do you have many storms like that?

"No, that was a real bad one. Don't have many like that."

"Well if you had answered that they were common, I'd have been off of this hill in a half hour, and set up where there is some low ground. Wow! That was scary!" (And not too bright! When we got to Wildwood the next week, we were told about lightning striking a tent the week we were at the Vineyard, killing two people who were in it.)

Monday Bud left for the city, we would not see him again as we would be leaving the Saturday he planned to be back.

"You boys have a good time and keep the water running."

"We will!" they chorused.

We made many trips to the beach for swimming and girl watching, but no connections were made.

Since this was a private beach, every beach trip required the presence of Betty. The beach was owned by another Eddy family (not related) from New Britain. There was an obvious implication (even we could sense) that going on that beach required Betty to be present if she had guests with her. Because of this, we went to the beach when Betty suggested it.

One day, Betty said, "Would you like to go with me to the Chilmark Exchange?" She had a huge smile on her face when she asked us.

"Sure. Sounds good to us," Jane answered.

Betty laughed and explained, "It's the town dump. We have gotten lots of furniture and other stuff from there over the years. If you take something down there because you don't want it any more and it is still good, you don't throw it in the dump, but leave it up top where the cars and trucks come in, so someone else can take it. Bud loves it and has even gone down to the bottom of the dump to salvage some things. I've seen whole sets of dishes carefully stacked by the road, old perfectly good beds, just anything imaginable. It's like Christmas when you go down there. You never know what you are going to find."

"Sounds like fun," I said. So we loaded up Betty's wagon with the rubbish and she headed down to the dump.

"Oh! Look at that!" she cried when she spotted a kitchen stool with steps that folded in under the seat. While it didn't look new, there wasn't a scratch on it. There was also an upright piano (!) sitting there (thoughtfully covered with a large piece of plastic sheeting to protect it from the elements 'til it found a new home.)

I stood at the top of the dump and looked down. There were old cars, tires, refrigerators, fifty-gallon drums, and more typical trash all tumbling down the hill to the bottom of a ravine. The gulls circling overhead testified to the presence of edible garbage, but it was not visible and there was no odor. After dumping our trash, Betty retrieved the kitchen stool, popped it into the back of the wagon, and we headed back home with our prize.

Next morning, when Betty could see activity on our hilltop, she called over from the kitchen steps of her hilltop: "Come see what I found in my mail box!" She was laughing.

I went over and observed that it was a seventeen pound striped bass. It was about thirty inches long, and getting it into a mailbox must have been a "grunt and shove." The silver stripes were what made me realize that this must be a famous "Striper."

"That's a nice looking fish," I said.

"Yes, isn't it? I found it in my mail box this morning," breathed Betty, "and do you know what else?" She smiled and looked at me in a way that made me wary.

"No. What?"

"I don't know how to clean them," she smiled.

"Neither do I!" I replied.

"Yes, but you're a surgeon!" She smiled triumphantly, and handed me a knife.

In the ensuing half hour, that seventeen pound bass went to an eating weight of around ten pounds at best. I started by amputating the head and the rear end, then I sliced open the fish from head end to rear end along the bottom. This let all sorts of entrails and organs come into view, which were quickly scraped into the pail holding the two ends of the fish.

All that was left was the body, but I seemed to remember that you had to scrape the scales off the body, so I proceeded to do that, going against the scales and they did come off. Hooray for me! At this point, I smelled like a fish, but I went into the kitchen where Betty had strategically kept out of my view, and handed her my project, proud as a fourth grader who had spelled "fish" correctly.

"Wonderful!" She enthused, "now you must all plan on coming to dinner tonight and we will enjoy it together. Why don't you all plan on being here at 5:30 so we can have some 'befores'?"

At 5:30 we were knocking at her kitchen door, and a cheery call came from within: "Come on in, and I hope you brought your appetites with you. Just help yourself to the hors d'oeuvres in the dining room, get yourself something to drink, and make your selves comfortable on the patio."

"The patio" was the front yard, and as we entered the dining room from the kitchen, I was astonished at the cleverness of Bud Eddy. The outside wall of the dining room was a Stanley roll up door! And in its open position, it allowed the room to merge into the yard overlooking the ocean. There were little tables and comfortable chairs placed around the patio area, which was limited by an old stone wall at its furthest point from the house.

The boys dove into the cheese dip and crackers and vegetable sticks (carrots, broccoli, and celery) and took their pick of the array of soft drinks. Betty, Jane, and I had some of the nibbles and joyfully consumed martinis on the rocks - with olives of course. (I could see that Betty and I had similar tastes, but Jane opted for a bourbon and ginger ale.)

Patches and Susie (Betty's youngest daughter) joined us for the evening and for the dinner. When the mosquitoes got too thick, we moved into the dining room, and Betty rolled down the door.

"Now everyone just take a place at the table, and I'll have the dinner on before you know it. I hope you're still hungry boys and girls."

With that, she disappeared into the kitchen, with Jane and Susie following her, and out came corn on the cob, fresh tomatoes, and my fish. Betty had stuffed it with spinach and baked it in the oven, and it was delicious.

"Gosh, Betty, this is a meal fit for a king! You went all out. Thank you," I said.

"Well Bob your talent at preparing the fish was really the important part. All the rest is just fresh-grown vegetables."

"I don't think I've ever had a fish that tasted so good. Your idea of stuffing it with spinach makes a huge difference in taste," Jane said.

When dinner was finished, the girls cleaned up and the boys excused themselves as they were playing hearts in the boat house.

Betty, Susie, Jane, and I adjourned to the living room, where yet another Eddy innovation was revealed to us. At about 9:30, Betty suggested to Susie that it was time for bed, so she said, "Okay, Mom." Then she gave her mom a kiss and said good night to us, turned to the wall in the living room and climbed up the ladder built between two two- by-fours that framed the room, and disappeared into a hole in the ceiling!

"Where's she going?" I asked.

Betty laughed. "Bud made the ladders for them. There are two bedrooms and a full bath up there. Bud thought the kids would enjoy the ladders in place of stairs."

"I'll be damned! How did he get the furniture up there?"

"He put it up there before he finished the floor. And some of the furniture came rom the Exchange." She chuckled.

"This has been quite a wonderful week with lots of new experiences. Thank you, Betty, for everything. We hate to leave, but we have to exchange boys Sunday."

Next morning we were up early, had had breakfast by eight, and broke camp in the next hour. When all was ready, I pointed the car down the hill and crashed through the brush and saplings, bouncing "baby" behind 'til I got to the gravel and dirt driveway. Once down, everyone piled in and we started out towards the road. When we got to the little gasoline pump for the house water, there was a call from the back seat. "We have to fill the drum on the roof before we leave," Dan called.

So while it filled, we all said our good byes again to Betty, thanking her once again. All the boys gave Patches a pat on the head and told Susie how much they had enjoyed being with her. She got all red as only a twelve-year-old can do, which caused an eruption of teasing from the boys, making the reddening worse, much to the delight of the boys. With water flowing down the roof, the car and "baby" eased out of the driveway onto the narrow road back to the ferry.

"Boy! That was a great week!" Kim said, and a chorus of "Yeahs" seconded his words.

We got home in about five hours after dropping off Kim. All dirty clothes were dropped in the back hall at the washing machine. Around five o'clock Jane said, "Let's have a pizza for supper. That way, I only have to get breakfast in the morning."

"Sounds good to me," I said. The boys were all for it, too.

Everyone headed for the showers, the first warm ones in a week, and how great that felt!

Next morning we repacked the clothes into the individual bags and put them back in "baby," drove over to pick up Carl Zimmerman, and, after a stop at McDonald's for breakfast, we were off to Wildwood, New Jersey.

It was a long five-hour ride on a very hot day. It seemed designed to have us broke by the time we got to our destination. There were toll booths over every hill and around every curve, plus the stink of heavy vehicle traffic and horrendous heat. Worst of all was the noise. Without air conditioning on a ninety-degree-day, the ride was one from hell.

Finally, we arrived at the campsite. It was separated from the ocean by a small local road, and the sites were located almost on top of each other. There was a shower and bathroom for females and one for males, right in the center of the tents. There was also the usual camp store where prices were at least double what they would be in a supermarket. Privacy was not to be had here. Sometimes the conversation in the next tent could be heard in its entirety. It was almost as bad as a public campground we had stayed in one night while on Prince

Edward Island. In that case our tent stakes overlapped the next tent and the conversation, all in French, never ceased. We left there the next morning.

The ocean here was the saving grace. Beautiful, three to four foot waves kept rolling in, and the water, fifty feet from shore, was only up to my thighs. It was the ideal set up for surfboards, and that was the first big expenditure; they were available for rent on the beach.

"Dad, can we rent some surfboards?" asked Peter, while the five other boys looked expectantly.

"Well let's see what they rent for."

"They're cheaper by the week, Dad," Dan said quickly.

So we had six surfers complete with boards for the entire week. The man who rented them fit the boys to different sizes depending on their height, and off they went full of ambition to "ride the curl."

For one week, Jane and I saw a lot of curls, with no one on them. We saw numerous attempts and subsequent splashes and heard a few choice words of frustration from the boys, especially when Finner, the littlest guy and just twelve, would surf by. Easily riding the board all the way to the beach, he would jump off as it scraped bottom, pick it up, and head back out, while the two oldest boys, Dan and Carl, struggled to get up and stay up, as he went by them, smiling.

A couple of times we took the night off from cooking and went to seafood places, and I'm here to tell you that six boys can eat a lot of lobster, given the opportunity.

"Boy this is great!" raved Finner. "I never had lobster before. It sure is good."

"Hey, Finner! You'd better not eat too much. You might not be able to get up on the board tomorrow," said a frustrated Zimmerman.

"I won't have any problem the way you guys are," replied the seventy-pound star.

It was truly a beach week, and the surfboards were a super success. By the end of the week, all of the boys were riding them; not as well as Finner, but enough so that they could say they had done it.

The trip home on Sunday was not as bad as the trip down. It was cooler, and we made good time getting home. We dropped Zimmerman off at his home. When we got to our house, we unloaded "baby" and then parked her in the garage until next year.

There is no question that we missed Jim dreadfully, but thanks to four great boys who came as our guests, and to Betty Eddy, the summer vacation was a great success.

I'm sure that both Jane and I felt his Jim's spirit and heard his laugh many times in that vacation.

PART 13:

SUMMIT ROAD

O ne night at about ten o'clock the phone rang. It was the answering service.

"Dr. Rackliffe, please call Mrs. Corvo as soon as possible. Her baby is vomiting."

The operator gave me the number, so I called Mrs. Corvo, thinking she was one of Dr. Greenblatt's patients.

"Hi, doc," a cheery voice answered. "This is Doris Corvo, and my children are patients of Dr. Z's, but he's not taking calls tonight, and Sue Mill suggested I call you."

"What seems to be the problem, Doris?" I asked.

"I have a six-week-old son who is vomiting every time I feed him. The doctor said it was colic and changed his formula, but he is no better at all."

"Is his vomitus colored, that is, does it look green or yellow?"

"Nope, doc, it's just white like milk." Her next sentence gave me the diagnosis. "When he vomits, it just shoots across the room."

"Think I'd better have a look. Where do you live?"

"I live at 98 Summit Road."

"I'm on my way," I said. I picked up my bag and headed for the door.

Summit Road was part of a new and beautiful low-income housing development, all Georgian-style brick condominiums, consisting of different size units. From one bedroom up to four bedrooms in size, they were tastefully arranged on serpentine roads so that speeding was impossible. There was a lot of green lawn around them, and there were several areas throughout the complex with playground equipment. It was just about six miles from the development where Jane and I lived.

After driving around a while, I finally found the right address and parked the car. I started up the sidewalk to the front door. As I reached the stoop, the door opened and I was greeted warmly by a short vivacious woman in her late twenties. She was holding the baby.

"I sure do thank you for coming doc," she said, as she led me into the living room. "Where do you want to look at him?"

"Why don't you sit down on the sofa and lay him across your lap?"

She complied, and as her husband Phil stood there watching, I examined the baby's ears, throat, and chest. He was obviously hungry, rooting around and looking for a nipple, at times sucking hungrily on his fist. Aside from the obvious hunger, all appeared normal, and importantly, he was not dehydrated.

I undid the baby's "onesie," and examined his abdomen, by gently putting my hand on the baby's stomach, pressing in the upper right part of it, and feeling for a little lump.

There it was! Diagnosis made.

"Tommy has an obstruction at the outlet of his stomach; nothing serious because you called before he got into trouble from dehydration. It's a condition called "Pyloric Stenosis, and peculiarly is usually found in first born sons. It is also inherited. The muscle at the outlet of the stomach (called the pylorus) is clamping down so that the milk can't get through into the intestines. He will have to have surgery, which is not difficult. The surgeon will go in and cut the circular muscle at the outlet of his stomach so that it can't clamp down as it is doing now."

"When does he have to have the surgery, doctor?" asked his dad.

"It would be better to get things started tonight, if possible."

"Okay, doc. Do you know a good surgeon?"

"I sure do. I'll call Dr. Bray to consult. He's great, a great guy and a super surgeon."

While they dressed the baby and changed their own clothes, I called and talked with George Bray and arranged to meet him in the emergency room in fifteen to twenty minutes. When the Corvos were ready I had them follow me to the hospital.

As we drove uphill through the park towards the hospital, we turned a corner to find the imposing building looming in the dark ahead of us, with the emergency area ablaze with lights and activity.

Phil followed me into the parking area and together the four of us went in the emergency entrance to find George standing there, already in scrubs. I introduced him to the Corvos.

"Happy to meet you both," he smiled as he shook Phil's hand. "Let's see what we have here."

He placed the baby on a gurney and gently felt his abdomen. Then he smiled.

"Well folks, it looks like Dr. Rackliffe is right on the diagnosis, but the good thing is that Tommy is in great shape for surgery. That won't take very long as it is a simple and very safe procedure, and there's nothing you have to worry about. What we'll do now is admit him, get some blood studies done tonight, and keep him hydrated with an IV drip. In the morning we will get x-rays to confirm the diagnosis and will plan on surgery tomorrow afternoon. Do you folks have any questions?"

Doris asked, "Will they put him to sleep?"

"Oh yes, and there will be an anesthesiologist managing his anesthesia during the surgery. He will be kept in the recovery room after surgery until he is fully awake."

The next day at noon, I went to the pediatric floor to see Doris to give her the news that the X-Rays confirmed the diagnosis, and that he was scheduled for surgery at 1:00 p.m.

"I'll be glad to get this over with, but I have to say that everyone has been so nice to us," she said. From the looks of the handkerchief she was twisting, she was plenty worried.

The orderlies came for Tommy at 12:50, and it was difficult to observe Doris watching him being wheeled away. She did walk with him out to the elevators.

"Mrs. Corvo, you will have to wait here. Dr. Bray will be up to see you as soon as the operation is over," the orderly said.

I could see Doris's lip quiver and her eyes fill with tears as she watched the gurney, with Tommy on it, roll into the elevator and the doors silently close.

I put my arm around her shoulders and said, "He'll be fine, Doris. Let's go down to the lobby snack shop and have a cup of coffee."

She welcomed the idea, and we had a light lunch along with the coffee. Then I went back to the office as she headed back up stairs to wait.

The surgery was over in an hour, and George was up there with the good news a few minutes after he had finished.

"Everything went fine in surgery, Doris. No problems at all," he said. "He should be on his way upstairs in about an hour. Tonight we will start him on clear liquid by mouth, and if he does well, we will start half strength formula in the morning."

Tommy was back in Doris's arms in about two hours after George's visit, took an ounce of sugar water without vomiting, and wanted more.

As planned, the baby nursed clear liquids that night, and in the morning he was given a half-strength formula, which he took hungrily again without any vomiting. The next day we gave him two bottles of regular formula, one at 7:00 a.m. and the next at 11:00 a.m. He wolfed them down and kept them down. Clearly, he was ready for discharge.

When I met Doris that morning at the hospital to give her final instructions, she listened intently, and when she understood all the instructions, she said, "There is something else I want to ask you about, doc."

"What's that?"

"Well, you know Phil and I are new in town, and we want to buy a house as soon as possible. Do you have any suggestions as to where we could find what we want in town?"

"Well you might want to look at Farmingdale. That's a new development where we live in a cape that has two bathrooms and four bedrooms. It is not fancy, but it's a new development, and a lot of nice young couples are buying there. The builders are putting up three types of house there; capes, split levels, and ranches."

"That sounds nice. What are they going for?"

When I told her the price, her eyes lit up, and I suspected that I had just met a new neighbor.

"Dr. Rackliffe, you are wanted in the emergency room right away. One of Dr. Vin's patients has been hit by a car and has a head injury. She is in the ER. Dr. Jim, the neurosurgeon, has already been called, and he asked that you meet him there." The no-nonsense voice from the answering service was curt. This was an urgent call.

I rushed up to greet Dr. Jim, who had already assessed the problem. He turned from the nurse when he saw me and smiled a tight little smile. "Hi, Bob, I could sure use your help with this one. Kelly was hit by a truck. She has a depressed fracture over her right cerebellar area. She is still in a coma, but her vital signs are steady. I want to operate right away."

He had ordered an operating room prepared.

Kelly was a ten-year-old, brown-haired girl who looked as Irish as her first name. She was in a deep coma. Her head was bleeding from the injury to the right rear part of the skull. There was an obvious depressed fracture, which could be seen through the gaping wound.

Dr. Jim spoke to the parents. "We have to take Kelly to surgery right away. The fractured bone is pressing on her brain, and may have lacerated it. We'll do the best we can, Mrs. Meehan, but we have no idea what we are going to find, or how badly damaged the brain is."

"Thank you, doctor," said Mrs. Meehan with tears in her eyes.

"There is a waiting room right outside the operating suite. You can wait there and I will see you as soon as we are done."

Jim and I went in to scrub, while nurses and technicians wheeled Kelly into the OR and placed her comatose body on the table. The anesthesiologist checked the IV line that had been started in the emergency room, while we prepped the area where we would be operating.

For the next three-plus hours, there was very little talking, just quiet commands. I assisted and marveled at Jim's skill. His fingers inside her skull assessed the damage. He carefully removed all that was not viable.

I assisted by suctioning the blood and debris out of his field of vision. We were both busy with clamps, shutting off bleeders as they came into view. Some of them we cauterized to stop the bleeding.

Eventually, Jim removed the entire right lobe of the cerebellum, which was damaged beyond repair. The lobe removed was the size of an orange.

The cerebellum gives us the ability to balance. It consists of two separate lobes, one on each side of the skull, in what are known as the Cerebellar fossa, and is located right next to the brainstem.

Finally, she was fixed as well as could be done. The depressed piece of bone was elevated and fitted against the skull, from where it had been broken. The covering layer was closed and the scalp sutured. Steroids were ordered to prevent swelling of the brain.

Steroids are very important as they prevent swelling of the brain after trauma as there is no room in a skull for a brain to swell. Indeed, severe swelling could kill her.

When Kelly was transferred from the OR to the recovery room, Jim and I went to see Mrs. Meehan, who was waiting anxiously for us.

"Mrs. Meehan, Kelly did fine in surgery, and is in the recovery room now. You can go in and sit with her after we finish talking," said Jim. "She has had a pretty large amount of damage to her cerebellum, but the rest of her brain is in good shape. Half of her cerebellum had to be removed. Now, this is the part of the brain that controls balance, so there may be some problems in that area, but you'll only know how much, if any, with time. Other than that, I'd say that she is going to be fine."

"Oh, thank you, doctor!" said Mrs. Meehan.

I walked out of the hospital with Jim. "Jim, I can't tell you how much I appreciate your being here and asking me to scrub with you."

"Hell, Bob, you did fine, and I thank you for helping. She'll probably come to in the next twenty-four to forty-eight hours, and then we'll know if she is truly going to be all right. Is she Vinny's patient?

"Yes. I'll have the service notify him in the morning, so he'll be following her, and you can bet I'll stick my head in there to see how she does."

Kelly was conscious late the next day, and her progress was rapid. Vinny and Jim had her walking with a cane by the end of the first week. She was a little unsteady, but I was amazed at her ability when I thought of that huge piece of brain that had been removed.

Within weeks, the Meehans filed suit against the truck driver and his company. I was not surprised then when about three years later, Doctor Vin called me and asked me if I remembered the case.

"I certainly do," I said. "Doctor Jim took half of her cerebellum the size of an orange out of her. How is she doing?"

"She's doing fine. The only residual effect is if she turns around fast, she has a problem with her balance. As you know, the parents sued the truck company whose truck had hit her. The insurance company that covers them hired the chief neurosurgeon of Hartford Hospital and another neurosurgeon, well known in Hartford, to testify in their favor that she is normal. Would you join me in testifying for Kelly?"

"Absolutely! She can't be normal after losing half of her cerebellum. I'd be glad to testify that I personally saw a piece of brain the size of an orange removed from her head."

The day of the trial (by jury), Vin and I drove up to the court in Hartford together. Vin was the first witness called, and what a charming speaker he was!

"Doctor Ringrose, are you familiar with the patient, Kelly Meehan?"

"Oh, indeed, I am, sir. I attended her birth and have taken care of her ever since." He smiled at the lawyer and the jury. "She has always been a sweetheart. You should see her step dance!"

"Will you give the court a little background on Kelly and this accident please, doctor?"

Vinnie's eyes sparkled as he turned to the jury and addressed them directly.

"Kelly, from the very start, was a beautiful and lovely child. She had an Irish temperament, that is to say, she was a happy child always laughing and happy, but she had a temper when irritated by something; she could put up a row. Again, like most Irish people, her angry spells were always over in a flash, and she would be laughing, step dancing, and playing with her brothers and sisters again. She was a great little help around the house, as most big families' children are. She was a delight to see when she came to the office, yes, a pure delight.

"Now I am here today for two reasons:

"1. To tell you what this adorable girl went through, and to report to you that Kelly made it through this horrible accident to be with us today; fortunately in fairly healthy condition.

"2. Now the second reason I am here is to emphasize the gravity and permanence of the injury to Kelly's brain. This was no minor bruise or bleed - oh no! This was a permanent change in her brain. My associate, Doctor Rackliffe, who is here today, assisted Dr. Collias that night and can testify to the degree of damage to Kelly's brain. Half of her cerebellum was so damaged that it had to be removed. That is, a piece of her brain the size of an orange was taken out."

He turned toward the jury as he said that, and emphasized the size so there could be no doubt in their minds. They looked at the beautiful child sitting there quietly, and many of them shook their heads.

"In the years since then Kelly has done remarkably well, showing steady progress towards normalcy, even doing Irish step dancing again." (Vinny gave the jury a huge Irish smile at that point.)

"However well she has done, and her progress has been very great, there are still issues. As the scar continues to tighten, we are concerned about her balance, and uncertain about her life and future."

As he blessed himself with the sign of the cross, he said, "It would not be surprising if she had seizures, which, thus far, thank God, she has not, but only time will tell.

"Through all the worry and fears of the last few years since the accident, the Meehans, fine family that they are, have been at her side. Mrs. Meehan gave up her job so that she could be home encouraging her and taking Kelly to the physical therapist, the neurologist, or me. Every time she came into my office, I could see slight improvement. She was a pleasure to see, and became more beautiful every year, and miraculously, appeared more normal each year. Her smile lights up my heart."

I was scheduled to go on the stand next, but at the end of Vinny's testimony; there was a hush in the courtroom as the defendant's attorneys asked for a brief recess.

They asked for the recess so they could discuss their options. Clearly Vinnie had impressed the jury with his presentation. As a result of Vinnie's testimony, the defendant's lawyers proposed a settlement substantially higher (three times higher) than their previous offer, and the case was settled right then and there.

In the fall of that year Doris Corvo called.

"Doc?"

"That's me," I answered. "What up?"

"Better call Dr. Bray again," she demanded "this one's got it, too"

"Got what?"

"Pyloric stenosis. He's hurlin' it across the room the same way as Tommie did."

She had had a second boy about five weeks earlier, and she was the kind of mother I trusted to give me honest appraisals. I knew if she saw it, it was there.

"Okay. Take him up to the emergency room and I'll call Dr. George." When I called George, he chuckled and said, "Okay, Bob work him up and let me know when I can go."

When I checked Jackie at the hospital he was a little dehydrated, but his electrolytes were okay. I ordered the x-rays which consisted of a barium swallow necessary to confirm the diagnosis.

Dr. Larkin, the hospital radiologist, called me, "Bob? This is John Larkin. Your patient baby Corvo has a positive "String Sign, so you can go ahead and operate on him."

The string sign simply meant that the outlet of the stomach was so constricted by the pyloric muscle that only a channel the size of a string got from the stomach into the intestines. This was in contrast to the normal channel of three-quarters to two inches.

With this confirmatory x-ray, I called George and said, "He's got the same thing as his brother, but his hydration is not where I would like it yet. Why don't you book him for surgery tomorrow?

Next morning, Jackie went down to surgery, and about an hour later, George called me.

"Bob? I just finished surgery on Jackie, and he's all set without any problem."

Mrs. Baker called on a Friday morning while I was in the office, and the receptionist put her right through, which meant trouble, and it was. She was in tears.

"What's the trouble, Marcia?"

"It's Phillip, doctor, and I need your help. He was hit by a hit-and-run driver and is in a coma at a hospital which she named nearer to her home. He has been there four days, and the brain wave has shown a flat line for the entire time. He's been on life support since we got there, and the surgeon says he is going to get better. He doesn't look to be any better, and some of the nurses and residents act as though they think he won't live. We don't know what to expect. What do you think we should do?"

Flat brain waves for four days sounded very much like he was actually dead, and I could not believe that a surgeon seeing that would be optimistic. "Marcia, you need to have another neurosurgeon see him in consultation, and I suggest you call Dr. Krause, who is also on the staff there, and ask him to see Phillip. Let me know what is going on."

I gave her Dr. Krause's number.

She called back in about three hours and said: "Dr. Krause is coming over here tomorrow morning at 10:00 a.m. to see Phillip."

"I'll be there too, Marcia."

Next day I got over there about 9:30 and went in to see Phillip, and to talk with the nurses who were taking care of Phillip.

"Is the EEG still flat?" I asked.

"Yes, doctor. Just like the last four days," one of them replied and shook her head sadly. "It's too bad, because he's been on life support too long now to allow the transplant team to use any of his organs."

Well! That was pretty definite evidence that the child was dead in the staff's opinion.

I had not been aware that there was a limited time for harvesting organs in those persons who were dead and on life support. That made his death even more tragic. Those kidneys and liver, and even his heart, might have saved someone else's child.

I went to sit with Marcia and Mr. Baker.

"What do you think, doctor?"

"He doesn't look good to me, Mr. Baker, but let's wait for Dr. Krause."

At precisely ten o'clock we heard heels clicking down the hallway, and Dr. Krause entered the room.

"Good morning. I am Dr. Krause, and you must be Mr. and Mrs. Baker." Looking at me, he asked, "And you?"

"I'm Bob Rackliffe, Phillip's pediatrician."

"I see." He turned to the Bakers and said, "I have examined your son, and I'm sorry to tell you that he is dead and has been for four days."

Just like that.

Mr. Baker asked the logical question. "If he has been dead for four days why did the other surgeon tell us he was going to be all right?"

The snappily dressed doctor looked stone-faced at the Bakers and said, "You'll have to ask him." With that, he turned on his heel and clicked out of the room.

I was stunned by his brusque, unfeeling manner, and his total disregard for the feelings of these two young parents who had been praying for good news, only to be treated like something stuck on his shoe.

This was at 10:45. I sat with them as they both sat there, weeping and silent.

Something had to be done. Finally I said to them as gently as I could, "It's now 10:45. At eleven o'clock, if you do not stop me, I am going out and check Phillip, and if there is no change, I am going to turn off the life support."

We sat there without speaking, and at eleven, I got up and said, "Unless you object, it is now time for me to go."

Their silence spoke eloquently.

I went into the room where the little guy lay, motors running, and an IV dripping. After looking over the charts, I spoke to the nurse in charge.

"Nurse, please discontinue life support for a moment, I wish to examine him after you have done so."

She nodded grimly and said, "Yes, doctor."

When all machines were stopped, I listened to Phillip's heart, and it was silent.

"I pronounce Phillip Baker dead. Please note the time, nurse."

"Yes, doctor." After she and the other nurse started disconnecting and removing all the tubes, she then combed his hair, and arranged his body so that he looked like he was sleeping.

I then went back to the room where the parents sat and said, "I have pronounced Phillip dead. I'm truly sorry. You can go see him now."

As one, they turned their tearful faces up to look at me and said, "Thank you, doctor."

That "Thank you, doctor" was because I had done something they could never have done; end the life of their son. It dawned on me then that this decision, in certain circumstances, was the responsibility of the physician.

The parents simply could not say those words. It behooves physicians to realize this fact when it occurs and ease the pain in hopeless conditions. Stepping up and taking the responsibility for the decision of life or death is part of being a doctor. Medicine is a science, but there is also an art of medicine. Too often decisions are made for legal considerations, rather than for the patients' needs and quality of life.

I remember when I first started my internship, I admitted a doctor who was in horrendous pain, as a dissecting aneurysm ripped apart his abdominal aorta. This was before the days when they could be repaired, and as I admitted him he said, "Doctor, I know I am going to die. All I ask of you is to control the pain."

"I promise you I will keep you free of pain, sir." I replied. I then ordered a quarter grain of morphine IV every four hours round the clock.

The nurses refused to give it (understandably since it was a lethal dose as ordered) so I got up every four hours at night to give him the morphine myself.

He died peacefully.

Again, my grandmother was in a convalescent home and suffering senile dementia. She was ninety two years old, when one night Dr. Scully called me to tell me that she had pneumonia. "What do you want to do, Bobbie?"

"Nothing, Roger, and thanks for the call."

He chuckled and said, "I thought you'd say that."

Pneumonia has always been called "the friend of the aged," and it is, unless in a case like my grandmother's, some damned fool doctor keeps her alive with antibiotics.

For what?

If death is inevitable, it should at least be painless. I recall another death of a family member who was in great pain during the act of dying.

A call was put in to the covering doctor, who refused to order any narcotic for this dying woman "because it was addictive"!

Duh.

About ten years after meeting and caring for Doris and her four children, they had moved into our neighborhood

We had made new friends. Phil, her husband, was a perfect mate for her. He worked at a local TV station and was obviously on the rise in that business. They were a lot of fun. Every encounter with that family was guaranteed to be interesting.

One Monday, Doris called for a house call for some reason or other. It was winter, so I went around to the kitchen door and rang the bell.

"Who is it?"

"It's Bob, Doris."

"Come around to the front door."

I thought that was a little weird because of the snow on the walks, but did as she commanded. I had to go down the driveway along the sidewalk and up the partially snow cleared entrance to the front door.

When Doris opened it, I could hear a lot of squealing and laughing coming from the hallway on the other side of the living room. Looking over Doris's shoulder, I could see there was a lot of action in the hallway. In addition, the kitchen table and all the kitchen chairs were in the living room.

I crossed the living room and looked at the scene in the kitchen and hallway. Each of the four kids (who were very small) had towels wrapped around their feet and they were skating up and down and around the hall and kitchen, laughing and shouting to each other as they slid by on the newly waxed linoleum, which shone like the floors of a convent.

I stood there and laughed at the sight, commenting to Doris, "Pretty sneaky way to get your floor cleaned."

"Can you think of a better way to polish a newly waxed floor?" she challenged.

A while later, Doris was pregnant again. Neither Doris nor Phil had any relatives living in the area. One day when she and Jane were having coffee, she mentioned this to Jane. Jane listened and then said, "Bob and I will be glad to take the two little ones for the three days you are in the hospital."

"Oh, that would be wonderful!" said Doris. "Sue Mill is going to take the older ones who can go to school with her kids."

This promise that was made when Doris was four months pregnant was promptly forgotten.

Later in the year, Jane and I went to a party at the country club, which turned into a raucous one when the drink of the night was introduced by Blair Beach. "I have a new drink for us tonight. It's called a 'Black

Russian,' and consists of equal parts vodka and Kahlua. Let's everyone have one."

It went down easily and hit hard, and nobody stopped at just one.

Next morning we were both awake in bed suffering alternating chills and sweats, headaches, and nausea. I can't recall any hangover being worse in my life. Neither of us wanted to do anything except take an Alka Seltzer and stay in bed.

The doorbell rang at eight o'clock.

I got up, put on my robe and staggered to the front door. I opened it and there was Phil holding two boys, in diapers, one in each hand, and each with a very thick, green, runny nose.

There was a big smile from the new dad, who looked exhausted.

"Here they are!" he said.

I looked at them with disbelief. The queasy feeling in my gut multiplied at least by five. I thought I was going to throw up.

There they stood, each with an obviously soaked diaper, smiling up at me.

I panicked. I looked at them in disbelief and hollered, "Jane! Phil is here with the kids. Doris had her baby!"

Then to Phil, "Come in, Phil. What did she have? Is everything okay?"

"Yeah, everything is fine. She had a little girl, and they are both doing well. I've got a load of stuff in the car for these two. I'll go get it."

Phil came back from the car with two suitcases, diapers, bottles (!!!!!!!!) and half dozen pacifiers. Jane took all the stuff and put it in the den. Then she changed their diapers.

How gallant and brave!

Phil left rather soon to go to the hospital. I had the feeling that after twenty-four hours of taking care of them, it was not so much to see Doris as it was to put some distance between himself and those two kids with their hygienic needs.

We made some coffee, and Jane set about taking care of those two urinating kids, who went through diapers like race cars on the final lap at the Indy 500.

I was happy to go to work in my peaceful office.

Another one of my families on Summit Road was the Bonzi family.

There were four children, two of them in diapers, and Florence, the mother, was a very reliable woman, whose opinion I trusted. When she called, it was never a nonsense call; someone was really sick. Every doctor has patients who are too quick to call, and others who are always too slow in calling.

Florence's calls were always justified. When I saw Florence's name on my list of calls one morning, I called her right back.

"Hi, Florence. This is Dr. Rackliffe. What's up?"

"Doc? I wonder if you could stop by today? I don't like the way Jackie is acting. He has a fever of 104."

"I'll try to get there this morning, Florence."

That summer day the temperature had to be in the nineties, and when I walked into her kitchen, Florence, who had two babies still in diapers, was washing diapers in her sink with a washboard and bucket. A washing machine stood in the corner of the kitchen.

I examined the sick child, whose problem was that he had a throat infection.

"I think this is viral, Florence. If you look over my shoulder, you can see little ulcers on the sides of the throat see?"

Florence stood behind me and looked.

"This is contagious, and some of your other kids will probably get it, too, in about a week. It doesn't require anything except time and Tylenol."

"That's good, doc. I can't afford any medicines right now."

Florence's money was frequently almost nil, since her gambling husband was not too steady at providing money and they had periods of real tough poverty, but he was a good man.

"Florence, why are you washing diapers with a washboard? What's the matter with that washing machine?" I pointed to it, standing in the corner.

"It's broken, doc."

"Well, why don't you get it fixed?"

"No money, doc."

I looked at her: ninety-eight pounds of skin and bones, and covered with sweat. It had to be over 100 degrees in that kitchen.

"Florence, call the repairman and have him fix it. He can send me the bill. You can't be expected to wash all those diapers and other clothes on a washboard with the temperature in the nineties or worse!"

At first she protested on the grounds that they owed me too much already, but she finally agreed, and I went on my way to my next house call. She called me that afternoon while I was in the office.

"Doc? This is Florence. The repairman will not fix the machine until he has your check. What'll I tell him?"

"Tell him to come and fix it tomorrow and a check will be there. How much does he want?"

"He said eighty-eight dollars."

"I'll stop by on the way home, Florence."

At least fifteen years later, Florence stormed into my office and asked to see me.

When she got to me, she stood there looking at me with tears in her eyes and said, "Doc, I am here to pay you all I owe you and to thank you for being so patient. I don't know what we would have done without you."

With that, she gave me a handful of 100 dollar bills, and then gave me a hug and a teary-eyed kiss. I had never expected to see that money again, and I didn't care. I had enjoyed the chance to do something for a lovely struggling woman. It pleased me that it was within my power to help someone like her. That was pay enough.

Florence was special. She was a woman of pure honesty and dignity, and the fact that she paid me for those years was just what I should have expected from a woman of such character. There was a lot of God in her.

Mary Kelaher also lived on Summit Road with her husband and *thirteen* children. I loved going there on a house call. It was always an orderly circus (and sometimes not). There was always a battle over who would carry my bag in from the car when I arrived.

All of Mrs. Kelaher's phone calls started the same way. She would say, "Good morning, doctor. If you happen to be over this way, Summit Road, would you mind stopping in?" This time she added, "I'm a bit concerned about Andrew, who has a bad cold and is complaining a wee bit about one ear."

"I think I can make it before lunch, Mary."

"Oh thank you, doctor."

When I arrived at their home, there would be shouts of, "The doctor's here!" and, as usual, before I could get all the way up the walk, one of the crew of thirteen kids would hurry out and take my bag with a huge Irish smile.

As I write this memoir, I am impressed by how much affection I have for the Irish. Most were friendly to a fault, non-judgmental, and genuinely happy people who showed their affection for each other.

Mrs. Kelaher, who didn't have an ounce of fat on her, was standing at the door with the sick child. She was smiling as I came up the walk.

We went into the living room with a gaggle of children trailing us to the sofa, where the first exam (of Andrew) took place, while he was surrounded by an open- mouthed horde of sisters and brothers waiting to see if Andrew was going to get a shot. (When that ever happened, they would stand transfixed with terror, and watch for the reaction from the victim.)

I looked into Andrew's ear to confirm Mary's diagnosis and let three or four of the siblings look in

"Eew! Gross!"

"Well, Mary, Andrew is going to need a prescription for that ear." So I wrote one out right then and there.

Then it started. (As it always did.)

From Mary, "While you're here, doc, would ye mind having a look at Marie? She's been saying her throat hurts but she hasn't had any fever."

I looked at Marie, whose throat looked fine.

"Doctor, Tim has been fussin' with a sliver in his foot; would you mind—"

The sliver was deftly removed by sliding it into a large needle, then bringing the needle out with the sliver inside it. (Just like I'd learned to do from one of the senior surgeons in town, who showed me this trick.)

And then Michael. "Mike, show the doctor the sore on your arm while he's here."

"Mike has a little impetigo here. Looks like he scratched a mosquito bite and got it infected. Scrub it with Dial soap, Mary, and put some triple antibiotic on it. Also Mike, you use a special wash cloth and towel that no one else will use."

"Yes, doctor," said Mike.

Then in a very soft voice, Mary said, "Would you mind looking at Claire's nipple—you boys get on out of here now! Hear me!!??" She sent all the boys out of the room. "It's all swollen and doesn't look right."

I looked at ten year old Claire (who was dying of embarrassment), and smiled. "Well, Mrs. Kelaher, Claire is becoming a lady and she's going to be a pretty one!"

Claire blushed.

"But doctor, it's only one side."

"That's okay, Mary. It often starts that way, but I guarantee you the other side will start, too."

After a few more "by the ways," I saw two or three more children, and then Mary showed me to the bathroom where there was a new bar of soap and a hand towel by the sink.

After my bag was all back together and I had washed my hands, I headed for the door (along with a flock of kids two of whom were carrying my bag). Mary stood by the door in a simple cotton dress with an apron on, clutching a well worn, small, brown snap purse and a big smile on her face. (I think at that time an in-city house call in the morning was seven dollars.)

"And how much will that be today, doctor?" she would say smiling at me with her purse clutched in both hands.

"Well, Mary. I think three dollars should cover it."

"God bless you, doctor." The purse would unsnap and out would come two one-dollar bills and four quarters.

As I left to go to the next house call, two little Irish boys ran ahead laughing and each one pulling on a handle of my bag.

"Goodbye, doctor!" they shouted and waved at me as I drove off.

PART 14:

CHANGES

I n my years in pediatric practice, out of five of
my families who lost a child, only two marriages
survived the trauma. With the exception of one
family, where the mother clearly blamed the father, I
could never understand why such a loss should drive
a wedge into what had been a loving relationship.

Sadly, the unexpected death of two loved ones hit
us in just ten days' time: first Jane's father unexpectedly,
and then our son. This was a tremendous blow for both
of us. Jane's reaction was to withdraw, to go into the
woods alone for long hours, attempting to come to grips
with what had befallen her. She bore her loss with the
stoic "old Yankee" thought of taking what comes your
way without showing emotion.

We accepted Jim's death, but never seemed able to
give solace to each other. When I told a psychologist
that we had not clung to each other in our moment of
agony, the reaction was disbelief. I don't recall ever having a discussion with Jane about the tragedy.

Meanwhile, the years moved on. In 1976, Peter married his high school sweetheart. They are a perfect match; both avid outdoors people. On their honeymoon they went to the Admiralty Islands off the coast of Alaska for two weeks, alone on one of the islands (except for the wildlife). A bush pilot flew them in and told them, "I'll pick you up in two weeks. By the way, do you have a rifle? There are grizzlies around here. Wear a bear bell if you go out to the bathroom at night."

They had no sooner gotten home from their honeymoon, when they headed out to Montana as fire wardens. Again, they were isolated on the shore of a lake in the Bitteroon Mountains, and had mice that became pets, along with a host of wild life that ranged from squirrels to moose and bears.

"I got into a situation where a moose got between me and the shore once," Peter told us with a smile. He didn't elaborate, but the thought was scary enough.

When they got home from that summer job, they turned right around and drove Pete's Toyota soft top to Washington state, where he enrolled for his Bachelor of Science degree, with an emphasis on math.

He ended up with a Master's degree in math from the University of New Hampshire, and started looking for a job as teacher. The school he liked had a huge outdoor program and was located in Maine. He applied and was turned down.

This was unacceptable to Peter. He asked to see the president again.

"I think you are making a mistake, sir. I am just what you need as a math teacher, with loads of camping experience and survival training. I would respectfully request that you at least give me a try."

The president looked at Peter over his granny glasses, smiled, and said, "I like your persistence let's do that."

Pete and his wife Vicki have been there ever since and have three children; the first born in 1977. All have finished college and are off starting the next generation.

Steve, the youngest, was the next to marry. He had graduated from the University of Massachusetts, and stayed on to get his Master's degree in Turf Sciences. He married Meg in June of 1980. At the time, he was green superintendent at Willimantic Country Club. As close to the University of Connecticut as it was, it was not surprising, given his credentials, that he eventually joined the faculty there to teach turf sciences. Steve and Meg have two children, both of whom have gone on for post-baccalaureate degrees as their parents had before them.

Dan, the oldest surviving son, served a hitch in the Navy. When he got out, he looked with interest on what Steve was doing, and decided that turf science and being a superintendent appealed to him, so he put himself through, refusing any help from us.

"I think I can handle this myself, Dad. Thanks anyway."

He not only did that, but he met and married his wife Jane, who is teaching Special Ed. They have three sons, all of whom are through college now.

Dan is a gentle soul, but I will never forget when he was only seven years old and we had just moved into our house on Lewis Road. He came tearing into the kitchen from outdoors in such a rush, I stopped him and asked, "What's going on?"

"Bobby Wallace is fighting with me."

I took him by the shoulder and turned him around, guiding him towards the door. "Go back out there and let him have it."

He was so angry at me, he went out and gave Bobby a thorough thrashing. From that day on, he never looked for a fight, but he never lost one either.

My boys always looked after each other, too. One time Peter threw a snowball at a boy much bigger and older than he was. His opponent was in the process of beating him, when Dan pulled Peter aside and took over for him. The opponent had a mouthful of expensive hardware which Danny managed to destroy in one blow. This cost our insurance company $750 in dental repairs. The agent sent Danny a letter praising him for standing up for his little brother, and finished the letter, "Please, Dan, don't be so thorough next time."

As a golf-course superintendent, Dan has written a book on the ideal golf-course repair building that treats the subject starting with bare ground, and finishes with a modern golf repair building, complete with all the equipment such a place demands.

During this time Jane's and my life together deteriorated. We both found it difficult to cope with the loss, and we couldn't find mutual comfort, which caused us to drift apart. We were cordial and did things such as golf together, and carried on an otherwise normal life, maintaining many friendships with other couples, as we had in the past.

Home alone however, things were different. Jane was very busy and involved in the state golf society and was away a lot playing in tournaments. I was happy that she was enjoying herself and keeping herself occupied.

Romantic or tender moments simply disappeared over time. That we ended up in divorce court was due to my infidelity −sad - but true.

The hardest part was telling my sons and their wives, but I arranged to visit each couple at their homes, and one by one, went to them and told them what was happening, and why. Both Peter and Steve expressed their displeasure at my behavior, while Dan and I discussed the possibility of reconciliation, since both Jane and I had each considered suicide briefly.

"Dan, reconciliation would never work. Forgiveness is not Jane's long point in this situation. She has already told me that 'I am as dead as my son,' so I see nothing to be gained by pursuing it."

"Okay, Dad," said Dan.

Now, all these years later, the families recognize and have come to terms with the situation.

This book is really about my experiences in medical practice and the events that happened along the way to that vocation, as amazing as they were unexpected, that helped me towards that goal. Jane was a huge factor in my getting through medical school, and her mother and father rank high on my list of wonderful people.

The events leading up to the divorce were certainly caused by me, but as a respected friend of Jane's father once said, "Dog poop doesn't smell unless you stir it." He was right, so as much as I regret the hurt that I caused, that is my own personal load to handle, and I prefer not to stir it anymore. However, precious memories will always be with me.

I moved out in the fall of 1987 into a two-room apartment, with a landlady who was a mother of three of my patients. It was in an apartment building in Plainville. When the movers came, Jane had left for the day, leaving a note to leave my garage door opener on the kitchen table.

The movers arrived and followed me around the house as I pointed out what to take. When all was in the truck, I moved my car outside, and after shutting the garage door, and leaving the opener on the kitchen table, I drove away from what had been my world for twenty-seven years.

My secretary Pat Daley helped me immensely in getting set up in my own home. I bought a water bed, which I had always wanted. It was wonderful to slide into its warmth and comfort, but water beds and cats don't mix too well.

Pat had also bought all the kitchen equipment, so I was ready to go. My furniture all came from The Pine Factory, and was rugged pine furniture plain, sturdy, and inexpensive.

Beverly was a single mom who I really got to know when her daughter Kristy (age seven) became ill. She had been going to another doctor in town and was not satisfied with the treatment she was getting for her sick child. A friend of hers who was a patient of mine recommended that she call me. She brought her daughter Kristy to the office that day, and she was very sick. After I finished my examination of her I said to Bev, "Your daughter has pneumonia, and I think she should be in the hospital."

"I don't have any hospital insurance but if that is what you want to do, I'll work it out somehow," she replied.

I looked at Kristy and asked, "Who takes care of her while you at work?" (She was an x-ray tech at the office in our building.)

"My mother."

"Well, if you can get her in here every day for me to see how she's doing, let's try keeping her home so you won't have that expense."

So we did it that way. In addition, I gave her enough samples that she did not have to buy a prescription.

Kristy did beautifully and was cured in about a week. At the end of the final visit Beverly pulled out her check book and said, "Thank you, Dr. Rackliffe. How much do I owe you?"

Now, this was a single mom not getting a cent of support from the child's father and working hard as well at being a mother. I just couldn't charge her anything, so I said to her, "Put away your checkbook, Beverly. We haven't done that much and you have enough to cope with. I couldn't take your money."

About a week went by, and a German coffee cake arrived at the office from Beverly.

It was delicious, and I made such a fuss over it. The first day, when I received it, I called her three times that day to tell her how good it was.

I think Bev thought I was weird, but I liked what I saw. She impressed me, and I found myself increasingly attracted to her.

I put a card on her windshield thanking her for the cake a week later and to my surprise and pleasure, a card showed up on my windshield a day or two after that.

What fun! The cards flew back and forth until I finally asked her out for our first date in January 1988. We went over to a restaurant in Waterbury, and it couldn't have been better. A barbershop quartet showed up after a contest in Hartford and sang the night away, while we enjoyed Caesar salad made at table side.

Bev was a joy to be with; quick-witted, patient, caring, and loving. Despite a significant difference in age, we were falling deeply in love.

We had some wonderful weekends staying at a friend's cottage on the beach in Charlestown, Rhode Island.

One night, there was a full moon, and Bev and I sat out on the deck looking at the ocean and the moon. The marsh in front of the porch waved gently in the evening breeze and the moon cast a soft light across it.

We spent about three hours looking at the moon, the ocean and listening to Chopin, Beethoven (Bev's favorite), and my favorite, Rachmaninoff. While we sat there listening, Bev asked me, "Bob, do you believe in God?"

"Absolutely! Despite the mess I've made of my marriage, I have felt and still feel that God has had a huge influence on my life. There have been too many strange coincidences for that not to be the case. What about you, Bev?"

"Oh yes! I have a lot of talks with him; I know that sounds funny, but I do. I was raised as a Catholic, but when I had some questions about things in the Bible, the priest told me that it was not for me to question, but to obey the priest's interpretation. That was unacceptable for me."

We talked about religion for a couple of hours before retiring. I liked the way Bev believed and I felt she really did have those conversations with God. In fact, she still does.

One night I invited Bev and Kristy over for dinner. Bev had said that she liked hot chili, so that night I served them Black Bart's Chili with a pear and walnut salad, and lots of saltines.

(Black Bart had a restaurant in New Britain, and he had a warning sign on the wall: "No one with a weak heart should eat my chili!")

"Phew! This is the hottest chili I ever ate!" exclaimed Bev. She literally broke out in a sweat!

I have to admit it was hot, but it tickled me to see her fanning herself from the heat it generated.

I asked her to marry me and when she agreed, I bought Kristy and her each an engagement ring. I wanted Kristy to know that we three were going to be a family.

A year later, Bev and I were married August 31, 1990, at the Redstone Hill Methodist Church in Plainville. My divorce had become final August 1, 1990.

My brother Foster was my best man, and Kristy (who was thirteen and beautiful) was the Maid of honor, while an older and dear friend, Sharon Pellegrino, was Bev's Matron of honor.

My brother's family was all there, as were my sister and her husband, and my brother Don and his wife. Don took on the job of photographer, and he got some great pictures. Bev's family was all there, too.

Bev looked beautiful as she walked down the aisle to a piano and violin rendition of Pachelbel Canon in D. The flowers on the altar were Bev's favorites, Stargazer lilies.

We had a wedding dinner at the Avon Old Farms Inn, and we honeymooned, with Kristy, at Green Hill Beach Motel, right on the Rhode Island shore. It was lovely.

Every day the weather was great. Our room had a small but functional kitchen, so we had breakfast in our room each day before heading down to the beach.

At night we went to various restaurants for sumptuous lobster, swordfish, or clam dinners, and reveled in each other's company. The first night I was surprised when Kristy ordered a lobster, and another of her favorites turned out to be calamari; very adult tastes for a young person.

We set up home in Farmington Chase, which is an assortment of private estates and condominiums beautifully set in a large grove of oaks. There are two tennis courts, a pool, and a clubhouse, too. The grounds are beautiful. We bought a two bedroom unit there and have lived there ever since.

When I returned to work, it seemed as though the practice had doubled, or else every one of my patients was sick at the same time. At that busy time I was on ward service, which meant that all admissions without insurance were assigned to my service.

That is how I ended up with Jimmy Marino.

Jimmy Marino was a ten-year-old boy who was playing on the train tracks behind his house with two of his friends, Johnny Garcia and Freddie Monroe. They were trying to run on one rail without falling off, and Johnnie was beating Jimmy with regularity. In the distance a train whistled, but Jimmy ignored it because he was having his best run ever, and didn't realize how close the train was. The other two boys yelled at him, but he was intent on his successful run.

When he looked up, the train was bearing down on him, brakes squealing, about 100 yards away. Jimmy froze in fear. He stared at the squealing locomotive and did not move. With a sickening thud, the train hurled the lad's body high in the air and forward, tossing his mangled body forward, where it fell entirely between the tracks.

When the train had passed over him, he lay there crumpled, still, unconscious and broken, with blood coming from his nose and mouth.

The medics were there within five minutes of the accident, and to their surprise, the boy was alive. They carefully put him on a back board and cleared the mucus and blood from his mouth, which improved his breathing so that they could take off for the hospital.

Arriving at the emergency room, he was wheeled into a small surgery where the ER doctor was waiting for him, having been forewarned that he was coming.

"Let's have him typed and cross matched for four units of blood right away, and get the x-ray team up here. We need chest, head, and right leg x-rays at once. Who's his doctor?"

"He's on ward service." That meant that Jimmy had no private doctor, so he would be cared for by the physicians and surgeons who had ward duty that month. That put him under the care of Dr. Joe Belkin for surgery, Dr. Dave Belman for orthopedics, and me for medical problems.

"His most pressing problem is the lung full of blood caused by the six broken ribs," Joe said. "Give him three of the units of blood as soon as they're available, and cross match him for four more," he ordered.

"Yes, doctor," said Karen, the nurse we were lucky to have assigned to Jimmy.

She was great!

"The skull x-rays show a crack but no depression," I said, after viewing the films. "He's pretty deep in coma, but stable, so we'll keep him on vital signs every hour for now." That meant we would monitor his pulse, blood pressure, respirations, pupils, and temperature hourly.

Meanwhile, Dr. Belman had attended to the fractured thigh, which along with the broken ribs, caused a severe loss of blood in the soft tissue of the thigh.

Joe made an incision over the area of the broken ribs and put a tube into the lung cavity running to a collecting bottle with underwater drainage. This allowed the lung to expand over time and for all the blood to drain out, replaced by the expanding lung, which was filling with air again. For the first two weeks, he lay there in coma without any response. The replacement of the blood lost in the lungs and broken femur helped stabilize him. But his coma was so deep that he just lay there. We fed him by tube and waited.

His condition was stable, but his coma was deep. Every day at least once, but usually twice, I would stick my finger into his clenched hand and say, "Jimmy! If you hear me, squeeze my finger!"

No response.

Every day it was the same, until he was in the fourth week of his coma, and when I asked him to squeeze my finger, he did! From then on, he responded more and more to commands.

One day I ordered him, "Jimmy, say hello."

After a moment his mouth moved. "Hello!"

From then on, he became increasingly able to speak and respond to questions.

One morning I asked him, "Jimmy, if you were playing on the railroad tracks and a train came along, what would you do?"

He didn't answer, so I said to him, "Jump! Now I'm going to ask you again. What would you do if you were on the railroad tracks and a train was coming?"

"Jump."

"Say it louder, Jimmy."

"Jump!"

From then on this was a question that started each day's conversation with him.

Over time he recovered all his faculties, and was back playing with the other kids on the ward and interacting with the nurses. He was everybody's favorite, with his friendly, smiley face. We had him in the hospital about two months, and we were all very happy to see his progress, and to finally see him go home healed and healthy.

When Jimmy was about fifteen, his mother called me: "Doctor, this is Mrs. Marino, Jimmy's mother. I am very worried about him. He is going around with some bad boys, and I think he is doing marijuana."

"Well, Mrs. Marino, we can't have that! I would like to see him in my office tomorrow night at five o'clock. I want to speak to him."

The next day, Jimmy was in the waiting room with his mother at five o'clock, and I summoned him in alone to my office.

"What the hell is going on with you, Jimmy? Your mother says you are going around with a bad group of boys, and she thinks you are doing marijuana. Is that right?"

"Only once or twice, Dr. Bob."

He was looking at the floor and shuffling his feet.

I put my hand under his chin, lifting it up so that we were looking into each other's eyes. He looked frightened.

"Well, you have to cut that out, do you hear me? Dr. Joe, Dr. Dave, and I worked too hard to keep you from dying for you to screw it all up! This pisses me off big time! Now I want your word that you will cut that kind of crap out! You're too good a kid to mess up like that, okay? You owe a lot of people who worked to keep you alive. You have to pay them back. Promise me you'll remember how hard everyone worked, so you could make it, okay?"

"Okay, Dr. Bob, I promise."

Jimmy kept his promise. He went to the local high school, where he became an excellent student, as well as getting involved in some of the clubs. He wanted to play football, but with his history of a fractured skull and the long coma from it, we nixed that idea and suggested tennis. He did pretty well with that and enjoyed the competition as a member of the school tennis team.

He had a host of friends. At graduation he took honors and received a scholarship for his first year in college. He was going places until one night a month before he was to leave for college; Jimmy and his girlfriend were driving home from a movie when a drunk driver ran a red light. Jimmy was crushed again, this time fatally.

Each spring for all those hospitals who have house staff and for all the graduating medical students, there is a period of great suspense. All the graduates register with the intern matching service, naming the hospital where they wish to serve their internship. Hospitals list those that they want first, too, but since there were never enough interns, most hospitals get fewer than they requested. Many hospitals accept foreign medical school graduates to help make up their house staff.

One year, New Britain General did not get one of the six interns they needed for the year. The residency slots were all filled (internal medicine, obstetrics and gynecology, and surgery), but no interns.

This posed a problem for the emergency room, as the need for interns was greatest there. To ensure that the ER was covered, the attending staff was ordered to each take a turn covering the emergency department for twenty-four hours. The selection was alphabetical and would require more than one day that year. Many of the older physicians hired residents from the nearby medical school to do their day for them, but most of the doctors in town took their turn themselves.

I chose to do my own service, too.

I arrived at 7:00 a.m. on my day to serve, had some coffee, and generally relaxed. I answered calls from my office and talked to my patients, having a few come up to the ER where they were seen by me. By agreement with the hospital, there was no hospital charge for seeing me at the hospital that day if they were my patients.

Mid morning, we were alerted by the police that there were some children being rushed in. They had been pulled out of a burning house on Bartlet Street. Apparently the father who was home with them had been unable to get them out.

Soon we could hear sirens getting closer. Shortly, a fireman in a yellow raincoat and boots came lumbering into the entrance, holding a small baby in his arms. He came right up to me and handed her to me. "Here, doc. See what you can do. I found her under the washing machine in the kitchen."

I looked at the baby of around twelve months. She was dead. Her skin was peeling off, and she looked like she had been roasted.

I shook my head and moved over to catch the next one as she was hurried in on a gurney by another yellow-slickered fireman.

This was another girl of about two years plus. She had second and third degree burns over about 50% of her body.

"I'll take care of this one," I said to the other doctors who had been called to help.

The two older children did not seem to be too badly burned. They had their burns dressed and went home with their mother and friends of the family.

My patient, on the other hand, was going to need minute-by-minute care. She needed someone with a knowledge of electrolyte and fluid balance, plasma expanders and wound management, all of which I was familiar with since I had been well-schooled in burn management during my residency. (Five years later

I wouldn't have had a clue, but right then I was the best in town for what was needed.) She was transferred to the pediatric ward, and she had everyone hopping for days. The care she got from the nurses was superb.

She was on the pediatric floor for weeks and became the spoiled favorite of the nurses who mothered her to the limit. Gifts and toys and candy treats were the order of the day every day.

She responded perfectly, and after several weeks went home. She became a patient of mine along with her older brother and sister for a few years, but then they moved away to a nearby town, and I lost all track of them.

I remember what her mother said to me the day she was discharged from the hospital. "I will never forget you, doctor. You saved my daughter's life."

And that was the truth, but it hadn't been just me. On my day in the ER I had been there for her. I had received help beyond imagining. My recall of burn management was surreal. I seemed to remember everything all of a sudden. I felt as if I was being guided, and in retrospect, I believe I was.

Those brave firemen, the entire ER staff, the lab people who ran chemistry and blood tests on her frequently to guide me in her needs almost hourly, and yes, God, saved her life.

Many times when the family would be in the office for some routine checkup I would look at her and smile. Seeing her made me feel good and I would experience a glow of satisfaction.

Twenty two years later, I had office hours on a Saturday morning, and the last appointment was a prenatal interview with a young couple expecting their first child (at any moment from the looks of things). She had lots of questions.

"How do you feel about breast feeding?" she asked.

"I encourage it emphatically. It's species specific, and all formulas are really attempts to duplicate it."

So we sat in the waiting room, and I answered all their questions as regards to my feelings on pacifiers (didn't matter to me, but a tough habit to break), introduction of foods (no hurry on that - after six months preferably), and so on for about an hour.

Finally, when they got up to leave, she thanked me for my time, opened the door and started out. She paused with her hand on the door knob and said, "By the way, doctor, does it mean anything if the baby hasn't moved in three days?"

I looked at her, startled by the question and disturbed by what it implied, since she was at term. Was the baby dead or was it in jeopardy with the umbilical cord around the neck?

"Sit down!" I said, "Who is your obstetrician?" She told me, and fortunately, I got hold of him right away. When he heard the story he said, "Have them go right up to the hospital, and I'll call ahead and have the surgical suite ready."

Three hours later, a baby girl was born alive, by caesarean section, with the cord around her neck two times. She was fine!

After finishing in the office, I went to examine the new arrival. She was perfect in every way, so then I went to see the mother.

"Your baby is absolutely perfect! Congratulations! What did you name her?"

"Victoria," she said.

"Shoulda named her Angela," I intoned.

The mother was the same girl I had treated for burns twenty years earlier.

PART 15:

HAITI

After my divorce and the closing of my practice in 1990, I became the physician for the New Britain School Board of Education, and when school was not in session, I started working part time for Dr. George Skarvinko in Southington. It was a large practice, consisting mostly of middle income families in a "bedroom" suburb. The practice was very well organized with an efficient and pleasant staff. The level of care was excellent, so when the school department did away with a full time physician in 1994, I joined the practice part time.

Because I was only in the office part time, I was free to do things outside of the office without causing any great inconvenience to the staff. The first opportunity to do something different came after I had been with George about two years.

I was playing golf one day with Don Amaro, a dentist from Norwich.

"Bob," he asked me on the third tee, "have you ever done any missionary medicine?"

This got my interest immediately. I had listened to my colleagues describing their missionary trips and had vowed that some day I was going to serve on one or two of them.

"No, I haven't," I answered, "have you?"

"Yes, I have. There is a dentist from Norwich, named Jeremiah Lowney, who has started a medical missionary program in the poorest part of Haiti. It's a town called Jeremie, which is on the western-most tip of the country."

I was impressed by the story that my friend told me about the Haitian Health Foundation, and what they were doing. After getting permission from Dr. Skarvinko to take the time off, I volunteered to go on the next trip. In addition to volunteering myself, I also volunteered Bev, since they had an x-ray machine down there. I thought she could help on that, as well as experience the entire mission, country, and people along with me.

I was so excited at the prospect of going to Haiti that I couldn't wait to tell Bev, and to ask her to go, too. A few nights later, while at home after working all day, I poured a couple of martinis, and told Bev about the upcoming trip. "I would like to go, and I would like you to come with me."

"That sounds like an interesting trip," she replied "I would like to do that, too." What a trooper!

The mission was scheduled in September for the coming month of January.

When January arrived, we had two duffel bags full of summer clothes and shoes that I had gotten from the people in our practice to be given to the Haitian children, and we were set to go. I also had gotten insulin that Dr. Lowney had told me was much needed. We met the rest of the contingent, including our leader (a dentist named Wilson), at Bradley Field and flew down to Miami. When we got to the gate for Haiti departure, there was a huge bright red sign from the U.S, State department warning all U.S. citizens not to go to Haiti, and if they did go, it was at their own risk.

We boarded the plane for Port-au-Prince, passing by the red sign as we did so. Dr. Wilson was carrying a much needed crankshaft for a Toyota with him.

As we touched down in Port-au-Prince, we were instructed to keep together when we disembarked, and to hang on tightly to our possessions.

Dr. Wilson told us, "We are supposed to meet a man named Oscar, who will guide us through the airport, so everyone please keep your eye out for him. He will be holding a sign with his name on it."

Once we found Oscar, he took us for our baggage, but we had to fight our way through very muscular men, all pushing and shoving to be near us. They were all trying to become our porters and carry our bundles, literally grabbing and trying to pull them out of our hands. Oscar shouted at them in Creole, and they backed off somewhat. We made our way to vans that took us to the extreme eastern end of the same airport. Here there was a smaller terminal for local planes. Everything was weighed, and we boarded a two-engine Russian-made transport for the flight from Port-au-Prince to Jeremie.

It was about an hour's ride to Jeremie, and once on course, with the cockpit door open, we could see both the pilot and the copilot were reading newspapers as we droned along.

All the emergency signs in this antique airplane were written in Russian. The airport we were heading for was a crushed coral airstrip under which the beheaded corpses of over a thousand mulattos were buried - killed on orders of "Papa Doc" Duvalier, because they were not "pure" Haitian. Ethnic cleansing.

The creaky old plane landed and taxied back over the coral burial grounds to a small airport terminal. This consisted of one room and two lavatories. As we disembarked, a single figure came out with a wheel barrow to unload all the bags and packages. Other men helped put it all into several waiting Toyota SUVs - the only car that could take the terrain, according to Dr. Lowney. Then the caravan finally started to the clinic on a coral road that presented one huge hole after another, making the ride to town a very bumpy one and making it necessary to go very slowly. The road was cut from the jungle and ran along the side of the hill with a fifty-to-one-hundred-foot drop to the ocean on the left side. There were beautiful beaches to be seen, but no easy way to get to them.

Finally, we came onto pavement and drove through a town that looked like a movie set for the beginning of the twentieth century.

There was a cobblestone street and broken down old buildings of concrete and wood that had not been touched by paint since their construction early in the twentieth century. People were everywhere. Many women and children were carrying large baskets, jugs, or bundles on their heads, often without holding on. The women looked regal as they strode along, magnificently erect, balancing the loads effortlessly. I did not see any men doing this; it was apparently a female task.

Electric wires were draped on crooked poles throughout the downtown. The shopkeepers had their wares on display on the ground. Such items as cloth, towels, and barrettes were right next to food stuff, such as fish, yams, turnips, and some fruits lying on the sidewalks in the sun. Flies were everywhere.

The whole area smelled. There was a mélange of odors, mostly on the pungent side. Oddly, despite the obvious poverty, everyone looked clean. Their white shirts were brilliantly white. All the school children wore spotlessly clean uniforms. The girls all had their hair in neat little braids held by colorful beads.

The village was right at the waterfront, but there was no fishing activity to be seen. There was a pier, but no boats visible. This puzzled me; for a starving people to ignore the food in the sea didn't make sense. The reason was that the Haitians had an inordinate fear of the water, and would not go out on a fishing boat.

We continued through the town on its cobblestone street (built by the Germans in the early 1900s) and turned a sharp right up a very steep hill. We passed a one-story building, which was the hospital for the town. A little further up, we came to a huge building of three stories, surrounded by a high wall with an entrance guarded by steel doors.

This was the Haitian Health Foundation, "Klinik Pep Bondyii," our home for the next week. It was an impressive structure. The entire compound was surrounded by an eight-foot cement wall with shards of glass embedded in the top of it, and barbed wire strung above that to discourage any unwanted visitors. The wall was about eighteen inches thick. All entries were equipped with steel gates that prevented any admission when closed.

The first or lowest floor of the building had a large door facing towards the road. This was the receiving room, used for the receipt of supplies and storage, as well as being the location for the batteries that were wired in to the entire building in case of electric power failure (a frequent occurrence).

The remainder of the first floor, fully half, was a computer room that contained the medical records of every person in every village (114 villages). (Incredibly, the level of compliance on vaccinations for children in those villages was greater than the level in the United States.)

The second floor had a library and conference rooms at one end, then an x-ray room where a donated x-ray machine from Hartford Hospital was run by a native who had been trained to operate it. Beside the pharmacy, there were about six examining rooms and two surgeries.

The third floor was the living area. On the land side of the building were several bedrooms, each with its own toilet, sink, and cold shower (there was no hot water, and the water was not potable). These rooms were about eight feet from the surrounding wall of the compound, and during the night we would occasionally hear the dogs under the window as they patrolled the compound.

On the ocean side of this floor from the dining room, there was a porch the entire length of the building, with a marble floor and comfortable chairs. It was to this area that everyone repaired at the end of the day, for some pleasant conversation, drinks, and snacks.

When dinner was announced, all would proceed into the dining room adjoining, and stand until grace would be said or sung. The evening meal would then be served.

At 6:30 the gates would be shut, and the guard dogs let out in the enclosed clinic. There were two or three German Shepherds and one Rottweiler.

Understandably, no one ever left the building until the dogs were back in their kennel area in the morning.

How did this clinic come to be?

Dr. Amaro filled me in on the background. "Dr. Lowney started his mission after he had been told that he had cancer and had six months to live. When he survived the six months, he figured he owed something to God, so he started coming down to Port-au-Prince every three months for a week each time. He would bring along anyone who wanted to come, be they medical, dental, or lay people who had skills. Together, they would help in any way they could, as many as they could, in this blighted city with raw sewage in the streets. These streets were dangerous to walk for fear of theft or injury.

"He aligned himself with Mother Teresa and pulled teeth, worked on oral tumors, anything he could do. One day, Mother Teresa came to Dr. Lowney and said, 'If you really want to do the most good, Jerry, you should set up your services in Jeremie, which is your name in Creole."

"The next trip down, Dr. Lowney and his group made their way to Jeremie and set up their clinic in an empty store in the downtown.

"After a couple of years in Jeremie, while he was scrubbing for a case at a Norwich Connecticut hospital, a surgeon approached him.

"'Hello, Dr. Lowney. I have been looking forward to meeting you and am so impressed with what you are doing in Haiti, which was my homeland before I became an American citizen.'

"'I'm pleased to meet you, too,' said Dr. Lowney. 'What was your home town?'

"'That's one of the reasons I've been anxious to meet you. My home town is Jeremie. I have some land there that you cannot buy because of the national laws, but I can give it to you, if you would like.'

"Dr. Lowney was delighted, and on his next trip to Haiti, he looked at the property, which was in the city, up on a hill. The whole piece was about seven acres in size. When he returned home, he notified the Haitian surgeon that he would be honored and privileged to accept the land."

Dr. Amaro continued, "After Dr. Lowney had received the land in Jeremie, he was talking to a very affluent friend about his dream of this clinic. The friend listened quietly, then asked, 'How much do you think this will cost?'

"About $450,000,' replied Dr. Lowney. The man got up, and using a pay phone, called his wife and talked with her for a while. Then he came back and sat down with Dr. Lowney, and said in soft voice, 'Jerry, build it. My wife and I will pay for it.'

"Next up was to consult with an architect to design a building to house the clinic. In addition, he started gathering people as a cadre to staff the program. He got the Franciscan nuns to manage the proposed building and care for the people, and a woman named Betty, who had a Ph.D. from the University of Connecticut, to organize a program to manage the health needs of 114 villages in the surrounding environs of Jeremie.

"The plan for the program was to hire a member of each village, pay them, and train them in the fundamentals of medical care. They were taught how to take blood pressure, give injections, listen to chests for pathology, treat dehydration orally with an electrolyte solution, and know when to refer to the nurse (there would be one nurse for every ten villages, all on the payroll of the Haitian Health Foundation).

"The nurses in turn, would refer to a physician employed and situated at the clinic, if they thought it necessary."

Dr. Amaro stopped and smiled: "Quite a man, eh?"

"A saint," was my reply.

On these missionary trips, we were required to pay for room and board and our transportation. In addition, everyone was asked to bring something for the cocktail hour, as well as any food you could manage to help feed the group. The specialty of the physicians who went on these trips was noted as well. If it was an ophthalmologist, Dr. Lowney brought in the people with eye problems from all the villages. When I was there, there was an abundance of sick children.

An interpreter was provided, and I was lucky to have the same man four out of five of my trips. He had a degree in law and a degree in nursing, but, for some reason, was unable to get accepted by the medical school in Haiti. He was excellent, and we became good friends. His name was Nestor, and he honored me one day by stopping at his home to introduce me to his wife, and stood by proudly as I examined his twenty-month-old son, who was a chubby, happy little boy.

Twice a week there would be a caravan of Toyotas going out to two of the 114 villages throughout the jungle. There were no roads, thus making an eight-mile-trip an hour or two away from the clinic. Five or six Toyota wagons would go on these trips with a pharmacy, dental equipment, including dental chairs, physicians, dentists, nurses, and lay people, who helped in all areas of the mission. Frequently on these trips, we would have to ford a rapidly moving river of clear shallow water that was about fifty to seventy-five feet wide. The bottom was covered with small smooth rocks, and each bank was covered with dark green shrubs. On both sides and in the water, there were Haitian women scrubbing clothes, and using lemons to bleach them white. There were women coming to the river with their baskets of clothes on their heads, and those who were finished, effortlessly swinging the huge baskets up onto their heads as they prepared to leave.

One of the trips was so long that we stopped in the jungle for a "bathroom break men to the rear and women to the front!" was the shout, and out we scrambled, happy for the chance.

In one village I was set up in a chicken coop, seeing the children on a table, with clucking chickens walking around amongst us as the clinic went on. Mostly the sicknesses were every day issues, such as ear infections, pneumonia, malaria, gastroenteritis, and skin diseases (lots of fungal problems).

There were some horrible things to see and treat as well. In one village a young mother brought in her seven-month-old baby, with a cloth covering the girl's head. Nestor told me that she had been told that "the baby doctor would fix her daughter." Nestor then asked her to remove the cloth, which she did, revealing a brain with no skull covering it. (This is caused by a failure of the neural tube to close during the development of the fetus.)

Failure to close is much more common at the buttocks end where that type of failure is called a meningocele. This child had an encephalocele (failure to close at the head end) the first and only one I have ever seen, and it was astounding to me that the child was still alive.

"Nestor, tell her I can't do anything for her, and that the child will die from an infection. But be sure to emphasize that this will not happen to her again. Any more babies will be fine."

This news understandably caused the mother to cry, and I was so moved by her agony that I put my arms around her and stood there for many minutes, me silently holding her, as she leaned against my shoulder and sobbed. I looked over at Nestor, and he had tears rolling down his cheeks as he watched us.

In this village we were in a room in the back of a church. Bev was outside helping, by doing fluoride treatments to the teeth of the children. Dental caries (tooth decay) was rampant, because it was a common practice amongst the natives, who were on the verge of starvation most of the time, to cut pieces of sugar cane and chew them. This destroyed their beautiful teeth quickly, to such a degree that dental caries was rampant. Sadly, the dental chairs brought along on these trips were not to repair teeth, but to remove them. The dentists were busy all the time we were visiting the village.

In the room in which I was working, I noticed a blackboard standing against the wall in a corner, covered with square root signs and equal signs from top to bottom. Along the bottom of the board there was a sentence: "Formula for finding the volume of a trapezoid." Who would have guessed, up here in the jungle.

"Nestor, what's this doing here? Who is doing this kind of math here?" I asked.

"There is a boy in this village who is fourteen years old. He does this," Nestor replied.

I have often wondered what ever happened to that brilliant boy.

That evening Sister Mary Ann took Bev and me into downtown Jeremie to show us the living quarters and buildings. A woman walked by, holding a young child with a drape over the child's face. Sister greeted her and asked her why she hadn't come back to the clinic.

The woman answered, "Because you didn't fix my child." With that, she took away the drape, and exposed the child's face. The right eyeball on this beautiful little girl was hanging, partially gangrenous, on the cheek. Sister Mary Ann took her the next day to see some visiting ophthalmologists, who were there from Emory University in Atlanta.

Arrangements were made so that within the month she was taken to Atlanta to have the eye removed, but she died within the year, due to its cancerous spread.

On my first trip to Jeremie, one of my first patients arrived, being held by a grandmother, riding on the back of a motorcycle, driven by a missionary preacher. They made their way into the examining room, with the tall thin preacher carrying the baby in his arms. He strode over to the table and quickly put the baby down, turned, and looked at me, "Phew! I didn't think we would make it! I thought he'd die on the way in."

I looked at the infant lying there. It looked to me like he wasn't far from it. He was blue and gasping. He was about five pounds (at three months of age!), dehydrated, and struggling for air.

His problem was in his mouth: he had the worst case of thrush I have ever seen, and because of it, he had not been able to nurse. He needed to be hospitalized with IV fluids. I told that to the volunteer nurse translator I was with that year, and she arranged to send him to the local hospital, along with orders written by me for IV fluids and care of the thrush.

At lunch time, she asked, "Would you like to go over to the hospital today when we finish here and check on the baby?"

"Yes, I would like that. He is so sick; I want to make sure that he gets what I ordered.

After we finished the afternoon clinic, the nurse and I went over to the hospital. That visit was an eye opener. The baby looked better, less dehydrated, but there was no IV going, just a lady sitting there with a thimble (!) getting fluids into the baby and it was working. The thrush looked as though they were successfully treating that, too.

My nurse translator then explained about the hospital. "It is staffed by Cuban physicians sent there by Fidel Castro. They get paid $37 a month, and there is a surgeon, anesthetist, internist, orthopedist, and a pediatrician. There is no food service here. Anyone who brings in a patient must supply the food as well and pay in advance for IV medications."

It was pretty humbling, seeing the baby improve by archaic methods, but rewarding that these people still had the ability to take care of their own, however primitively.

I found the Cuban doctors to be well-trained and capable, and very friendly.

Occasionally they were invited to dinner at the clinic when there was enough special food of higher quality than usual. For example, pork loins that Bev and I brought down one year were never seen by our group of volunteers. Instead, they were served to the Cuban doctors and some high ranking politically helpful visitors from the states.

Meal times were always preceded by a song or grace before the meal. Seating was never the same two nights in a row, as everyone mixed well and wanted to talk to others about their day.

Almost everyone was in bed by nine. The dogs were let out of their cage at six p.m., right after the main gate was closed. During the night we could hear the dogs go by our bedroom window, patrolling the grounds and the walls, which also had glass shards embedded in the cement on the top. Security was no joke here. People were often desperate for food.

Whenever we went into Jeremie to do shopping or to visit some sick person, there would always be a crowd of little children begging for money, gum, candy or something we were wearing (bracelets, watches, earrings, and any thing else they saw). There were a few dogs whose main food supply was the rats, which were pretty brazen, often nibbling on sleeping people. Strangely, I never saw a cat.

I wondered if the huge loads carried on the heads of these tall, graceful, regal- looking women caused any long-term medical problems with their necks. The local doctor said they did not.

The vast majority of the people lived in two-room cement-sided and floored houses, with metal corrugated roofs. In one room was a box slightly bigger than a double bed. It was raised on legs to a height of about twelve inches. At bedtime, the whole family would remove their clothes, spread them around in the box and then all would climb in for the night! Mother, father, children— all of them.

On the third day of my first visit to Haiti, I was just finishing the morning work at the clinic with my interpreter, a French Canadian nurse named Colette, when a very pretty and smiling young nun from India appeared, wearing the same habit as Mother Teresa. She and Colette talked for a minute and then Colette turned to me.

"This is Sister Saari. She is from Mother Teresa's orphanage in town here and she heard there was a baby doctor here this week. She wants to know if you could come down and see a few of their children that they are worried about."

"Of course, but I didn't know that Mother Teresa had an orphanage here."

"Yes. It is actually an orphanage and a hospital for people dying of AIDS. There are two wings to the building, the hospital in one, and the orphanage in the other. We should be through here by three. Would you like to go then?"

"That will be fine."

At the same time we were ready to go, Bev was through with her work, and I invited her to come along.

The orphanage was really a short distance from the clinic, and as we drove up we could see a guard outside the gated entrance. We parked in the street, and as we walked toward the entrance we saw Sister Saari smiling and walking toward us to welcome us at the gate. Upon entering, we were surrounded by hordes of little children, of ages two to five, wearing shirts and shorts, and no shoes.

The building and the playground were entirely concrete. In the playground there was a drain in the center and a hose at one end, which explained why it looked clean. Toys were sparse; a few large balls, plastic buckets, and not much else.

Sister Saari guided us into the dormitory in the front of the building. It was a room of about fifty feet in length and thirty-five feet in width. It contained thirty or forty cast iron cribs, vintage 1900, all the same size; forty by twenty-five inches. Each crib had a thin rubber foam mattress and no sheets.

Sister guided me to one with a screaming infant in it. The baby had good cause to scream. He had a terrible ear infection. I prescribed some antibiotic to Colette, who transmitted the information to the sister, who smiled and nodded.

The remainder of the children I saw had minor things, like infected wounds or scratches, fungal infections of the skin, and one newcomer, an infant of eight months, who weighed at just eight to ten pounds. All he needed was food.

While I was examining all these little ones, Bev had noticed a little girl of about three who kept to herself, away from the other children, and kept staring at Bev. She ignored the other children completely and kept lingering near Bev.

Bev approached her, combed her hair, and talked to her, although neither could understand what was being said. Pretty soon, Bev was holding her, and the little girl snuggled into Bev's neck, repeatedly saying, "Mama."

We went outside with Sister and watched twelve little ones get washed. Two more Indian sisters lined them up behind the orphanage on some grass. Then the children undressed, and laid their clothes on the ground before stepping back to a little trench. Sister Saari then hosed them all down with cold water, which wasn't very cold, and the other two started down both sides of the children, soaping them from top to bottom. Sister Saari followed behind, rinsing off the squealing children. Then they put their clothes back on, wet as they were.

As we got ready to go, Bev had to put the little girl down and tried to get her to wave without success.

We returned to the clinic and prepared for the social hour. Bev was very quiet all evening. When we retired for the evening, she suggested we sit on the porch for a while. I sat there, just enjoying the evening air, and watching the bats flying around in the floodlighted areas.

Finally Bev spoke, "Bob, would you mind if we adopted that little girl?" She had tears in her eyes.

"Of course not. We'll go back tomorrow and see the Mother Superior."

"Oh, that's wonderful! I was afraid you would say no. She is such a sweet little girl, and she loved being held and fussed over. Poor little thing, she needs a mother."

The next afternoon, Bev and I were taken over to the orphanage by one of the drivers. When we got there, I asked to see the Mother Superior.

An older nun in the same habit as Mother Teresa came toward us smiling.

"Hello, doctor, did you want to see me?"

"Yes, Mother, may I introduce my wife Beverly?"

The two women shook hands and smiled at each other.

"What can I do for you?" asked the nun.

"We would like to adopt one of the little ones we saw here yesterday. Is that possible?"

The nun's smile faded. She paused and then said very sadly, "Oh no. None of these children are up for adoption. They are left here without anyone ever seeing their parents. They are here because their parents cannot feed them, but they might come at any time and take them back. This orphanage is always being watched so that the children here will not be taken away. At any moment of any day, a car may drive up and stop in front of our guard and have a child handed to him. No words are said, and we then have another child to care for.

"If you would like to adopt a child, you must go to Port-au-Prince to the orphanage there, and of course, you must be Catholic."

Crushed, I thanked her for seeing us and as we left sadly, Bev saw her little girl looking at us, and she waved at Bev. The wave was returned through teary eyes.

The next year Bev brought with her a little gold necklace, in case the girl was still there. She was and ran to Bev immediately. The two of them hugged, and Bev was in tears as she examined her little girl to be sure she was all right. She put the necklace around her neck and kissed her.

When it time came to go, Bev picked up the little girl. As she snuggled into Bev's neck and kissed her, she again said, "Mama."

Bev kissed her back and we left, both of us in tears by this time.

"I'm never coming back here again," Bev said, "it's just cruel to love someone as I do her and she does me, and not be able to be together. Especially when nobody else wants her."

On our later trips Bev never went back to the orphanage, but I went back one or two times in later years, and the little girl was still there. The necklace was gone.

On another of our trips, the nuns who ran the clinic asked me if I would "mind" doing some physicals at a Protestant orphanage. Being Protestant, we found this amusing. Bev and I agreed to go.

I should tell you that Bev had worked in an orthopedic hospital for children in Newington, Connecticut, and probably knew more about orthopedic deformities in children than I did. Because of that, when we were examining the children, Bev leaned over to me, as the next child was advancing to be examined, and whispered in my ear, "This next little girl has a congenital dislocation of her left hip. I can tell because of the way she walks."

I would not have picked up on this, because I was examining the child who preceded her, and did not see her walk. But having been forewarned by Bev, I tried to rotate her left leg internally while it was flexed, and sure enough, it could not be done, confirming Bev's diagnosis.

I asked if the orphanage had the ability or where-withal to have this darling little four-year-old's problem attended to, and they assured me that they did, so there is one little Haitian girl walking normally, thanks to the sharp eyes of my wife.

Building concrete houses of two rooms and a corrugated roof was a project of the Haitian Health foundation. They were building them for the Haitians as quickly as they could get the money; in donations from interested people, churches, and service clubs such as Rotary, Kiwanis, and the Lions.

We saw other homes that were made of cloth and sticks with dirt floors.

Two more of the foundation's projects were to restore the chicken and pig population, which had been decimated by epidemics and probably further stressed by the starving population.

One of the nuns at the clinic, Sister Mary Mac, had a clutch of rabbits she was raising – a- suitable choice of food for the natives, and given a chance to start to reproduce, could multiply rapidly.

In Jeremie, there are two demanding and critical problems that need addressing. One is "Kwashiorkor," a disease caused by protein deficiency. It is rampant on the island, and demands action. Children afflicted with this disease are bloated, and have red sparse hair. They are weak and in desperate straits, demanding IV hydration and protein supplements. The worst ones need to be hospitalized, or they will die.

The second urgent problem is toxemia of pregnancy, which can cause elevated blood pressure, convulsions, and death if not treated at once. The lack of roads prevented quick lifesaving treatment. It took too long to get to the clinic from a village ten miles away. Dr. Lowney and his nursing staff set about on the gigantic task of building a hospital in town, where they could bring in the eclamptic women and the severe Kwashiorkor cases to monitor them day and night.

Sister Mary Ann, the head nurse and the top person at the clinic, started looking for land near the clinic. The land had to be large enough to establish living quarters, a hospital, and a pavilion to be used for teaching. There would also have to be room for a vault-like building in which to safely store food stuffs. These donations came in huge quantities by companies and the U.S. government, as well as service groups and churches. She located a splendid area for the new campus, about ten acres and fairly close to the clinic. It was owned by a Haitian by the name of Phillipe Boutot.

Sister Mary Ann went to see him.

"Monsieur Boutot, I am Sister Mary Ann of the clinic, and I would like buy your land over near the clinic," she said.

"Oh yes, Sister! That is a very fine piece of land, and as it happens, it is for sale at a very fair price," Monsieur Boutot responded eagerly.

"And what would that price be?" asked the good sister.

"Sixty thousand dollars, which includes all twelve acres and the buildings on them," he replied.

"Oh!" gasped Sister Mary Ann. "that is much too dear. We cannot afford that, but I thank you for your time," she said, as she bid him good bye.

About two weeks later, Monsieur Boutot came to the clinic to see Sister Mary Ann.

"It's good to see you again Monsieur Boutot. What can I do for you?" smiled the nun, knowing full well another offer was going to be presented.

"Well, Sister, I have been thinking of all the good you do here in Jeremie, so I have decided to really make you a most generous offer for the parcel of land."

"And what would that be?" Sister Mary Ann asked, demurely.

"I have decided to offer it to you for thirty five thousand dollars; you can appreciate what a generous offer this is, Sister."

"I appreciate your offer, Mr. Boutot, but it is still above the price the clinic can afford," replied Sister, and then she added, "How old are you, Monsieur Boutot?"

"I am in my mid-sixties, Sister. Why do you ask?"

"Well, you know you are getting up there to the age when …" Sister left the sentence unfinished, and then continued: "I want you to know, Monsieur Boutot, that I will pray for you every night that you may go to Heaven when you die. Thank you for the generous reduction in price, and I only wish we could afford it." Speaking thus, she ended the conversation, and Monsieur Boutot left the clinic with much sadness to ponder what Sister had said.

Ten days later, Monsieur Boutot reappeared at the clinic and asked to see Sister Mary Ann. He was carrying a rolled up piece of paper.

"Bonjour Monsieur Boutot. How are you today and what brings you here?" Sister Mary Ann greeted him.

"I have come to make my final offer, and I have with me the title to show you what I paid for the land you desire. I am asking you to pay twenty-two thousand dollars, which, as you can see, is just two thousand more than I paid for it."

Sister Mary Ann studied the title, and found that Monsieur Boutot was telling the truth. "That's very generous, Monsieur Boutot. If you will give me a minute I will call Dr. Lowney to see if this is acceptable to him."

She then called Dr. Lowney in the states and gave him the news, asking him what he would like to do.

"Buy it, Sister."

She then returned to the room where Monsieur Boutot was waiting and said, " Monsieur Boutot, we thank you for the offer, and we will accept it."

"That is wonderful Sister! I am very happy now. There is one thing more though, Sister."

"What is that?"

"Will you please stop praying for me? I haven't had a good night's sleep since you started!"

Sister laughed and reassured him that she would think only good things about him and his generosity. "I think, Monsieur Boutot that you will live a long time more, and you needn't worry about the future."

The next year a volunteer engineer and his wife came from France to do the building. With hordes of local laborers, a twenty-four bed hospital was erected on one level, cleverly illuminated with glass brick. There is a veranda all around the front and two sides. In addition, two three-story homes of European design were completely refurbished and provided the staff with decent apartments.

A large pavilion was constructed, as well as a thief-proof huge hexagonal storage building, where the foodstuff was safely stored. It was concrete up to the roof, which was supported by eight-by-six beams, bolted down on the inside. There would be no thieves, either four-legged or two-legged in there. The French couple stayed on until they had finished building the new campus. The engineer's wife jumped in to help treat the patients at the clinic and assist in any other way that was needed.

There are twelve beds for children with Kwashiorkor, and twelve beds for the high risk pregnancies in the little hospital that will save many lives. All the surgical equipment needed, along with two operating tables, were contributed by the New Britain General Hospital in New Britain, Connecticut.

There was also a pavilion constructed adjacent to the food storage unit, and was about one hundred feet long and sixty feet wide. Inside, there were chairs and a baby scale, which was actually a large fish scale, hanging from the crossbeam, hooked on to a canvas hammock, supporting the baby being weighed. On the outskirts of the pavilion, there were many brightly painted child-size chairs and tables, some of which this old doc had helped to paint.

This pavilion was used to teach the mothers about nutrition, especially emphasizing breast feeding, telling them how to treat diarrhea and pneumonia, all by songs. They had to learn these songs and sing them in order to get their monthly allotment of grain and a pint of cooking oil. It was pure bribery, but effective.

This pavilion was also where I saw sick children. I was seated with an interpreter at the table, with the mothers and patients in line, waiting their turn. I counted sixty before I was done.

The very last patient had an infected ear, for which I prescribed some antibiotic, and assumed we were through, when the mother opened her shirt, exposing her breast, and asked through the interpreter, "What about this?"

"This" was a hard mass in the upper inner part of her left breast. The mass was rock hard, but freely moveable and about two inches in circumference. I first thought it was an abscess and instructed her to come to clinic in the morning, when I planned on opening and draining it.

Next morning, I saw her again and reassessed the mass. It was not tender, nor could I detect any fluid.

My conclusion was, it was not an abscess, but probably cancer. Coming to that decision, I referred her to the hospital for the Cuban surgeon to see. This meant that her stay there and the responsibility to feed her would rest with the Haitian Health Foundation. So be it.

At the end of our week at the clinic and villages, we arose on the seventh day, had our last breakfast with the three sisters, and proceeded to the local airport. When the old Russian plane arrived, our luggage was put aboard after being wheeled to the plane in the wheel barrow. We waved our good byes and buckled in as the old junk trundled down for takeoff over the thousand beheaded Haitians. Shaking and rattling, it zoomed down the coral strip and into the air towards Port-au-Prince.

The transfer from the local terminal to the international terminal at the other end of the same runway was a fight to keep our luggage in our own hands again, as it had been on arrival. Finally we were in line to depart, and after checking our luggage in for the flight home and passing through security, we were finally free of the pushing, shoving mobs.

As we sat in the restaurant waiting to board our plane for the flight home, Bev started to cry.

"Why are you crying?" I asked.

"Because I am never going to be like I've been this week again. I've been just me, helping and loving, with no expectations or demands, no past history, nothing but me. It's been wonderful."

We spent some time in a restaurant waiting to board, finally walking out to the plane, and climbing the stairs to be welcomed aboard.

I must confess a feeling of relief and safety came over me as I settled into my seat in delightfully cool air conditioned comfort heading home.

Upon arrival in Miami, Bev and I made our way to the gate for Bradley Field, and after getting a couple of sodas, sat down to await the departure. I was chatting with Bev when I felt a thump on my left foot. Looking up I saw Al and his wife Nancy, who were members of my country club back home.

"Where are you coming from?" asked Al.

"Haiti," I replied.

"I didn't know they had golf courses there," he said.

"They don't. Bev and I were on a medical missionary trip."

'Oh."

"How wonderful!" his wife exclaimed, "I'll bet that was interesting!"

Before I could respond, Al walked away. No golf, no interest.

Within three minutes of their departure, another couple from the club came into view, and seeing us sitting there, came over to chat.

"Hi, Bob, and this must be Bev," Bertha greeted us. This was the first time she had met Bev, but she certainly had heard of her.

"Where have you two been?" we inquired.

"We are on our way home from a Club Med, and we had a wonderful time. How about you two?"

"We have been in Haiti for a week on a medical mission," I replied.

"How wonderful! Would you be willing to give a talk on your experiences to my Woman's Club? I'm sure it would be interesting to hear about the challenges and life there."

"I'd be delighted. Just give me a call."

They walked away as Al and Nancy had, as though they were caught with a hand in the cookie jar, which amused both Bev and me.

Bev and I have had our share of vacations to lovely places, but as Bev said, "This week in Haiti has meant so much more to me, to see the need of these lovely, proud, people and to be able to help them is just so gratifying. I don't ever recall coming home from a vacation feeling so fulfilled, so content."

I felt the same way.

Getting back into the swing of practice in Southington was almost ludicrous. After seeing up to sixty really sick patients per day for six days, to drop down to routine physicals, runny noses, feeding problems (not in Haiti! where the only feeding problem was to find formula), earaches, and mostly unsick children was nowhere near as satisfying or challenging.

In October 2006, the partner who was working part time resigned from the partnership. The replacement physician was hired for full-time work. That made my part- time position unnecessary, thus ending my employment.

The time had come to sit back, enjoy life, and volunteer my time for needy projects or people. Physical limitations have impacted my usefulness in that regard, however.

Every now and then, much to my joy, I keep bumping into parents or children of my practice years. It's so gratifying to see and hear of their successes in life and to feel the warm affection they share with me for our relationship.

One of my babies is now a practicing pediatrician in the group that I started with Harold in 1956. That makes me feel very proud!

My main goal when I started out was, like George and I promised on the jungle road of Saipan, to serve God by serving my fellow man. What I hadn't expected was that giving to my patients, and loving them, was a gift that would be returned tenfold. My practice years were full of gestures and acts of affection from both my patients and their parents.

I thank God whose presence I have felt so many times, who had arranged for my education and for the opportunities to serve him, I thank him for the inspiration given to me by George Radford DVM.

I remember reading these words whose writer is unknown to me, early on in my practice:

"Lord, save for those who are old and rougher, the things that little children suffer."

Amen.

ACKNOWLEDGEMENTS

I am deeply indebted to my niece, Kathy Cox and Dr. Gerry Neipp, both published authors, for their unselfish and almost constant help at the outset of my effort. My friend Joanne Spence, an expert grammarian who proof read the whole work and corrected the many errors, was always smiling and willing to look at a problematical sentence or paragraph and fix it.

A dear friend in the U.K., also a published author, my ever helpful Peter Dowles guided me through computer problems and suggested ways to make a point that never would have occurred to me.

And finally, by sheer accident,(?) I mentioned to my friend Malo Forde that I was writing a book. This lead to another "coincidence" that God put in place to help me chapter by chapter and word for word get this book written the way it should be read and leave the reader with the knowledge that: *Nothing is impossible.*

Made in the USA
Lexington, KY
05 September 2011